TALES AND TRAVELS OF AN EXPEDITION DOCTOR

Happy journey to safer places!

Bill

TALES AND TRAVELS OF AN EXPEDITION DOCTOR

William J Turner MB CLB

TEMPLE

TEMPLE PUBLISHING COMPANY
London, England

First published in Great Britain 1995
by Temple Press
London, England

Reprinted 1995

**British Library Cataloguing-in-Publication Data.
A catalogue record for this book is available
from the British Library**

ISBN 1 85977 000 2

Cover design by Harold King

Printed & bound in England by
Antony Rowe Ltd, Chippenham, Wiltshire

CONTENTS

INTRODUCTION

I qualified at medical school in Liverpool in 1968 and after a short spell in hospital entered general practice where I have remained for the last twenty years. I have always been interested in hill walking and travel. The Lake District, North Wales and especially Scotland were always popular haunts for me. The outdoor life, the wind, the weather and mountains have always fascinated me.

My first contact with expedition medicine was by accident. I decided with a friend to walk the Pennine way and contacted the then Managing Director of Karrimor for information about equipment. To our surprise, he invited us out to dinner to meet a Commissioner of Scouts who was looking for doctors to help him on his expeditions. That is how I met Peter Drake.

Peter was raised in South Africa and spent his formative years there before coming back to England. A man with expeditions and adventure in his blood. Having met Peter since 1975 he has shown me sights I would otherwise never ever have seen. He has introduced me either intentionally or by accident to people I will never forget and has put me in situations which I will never forget, nor sometimes forgive. But for all those memories and many more I will always be extremely grateful to him. Wherever he leads I would follow and that is an extremely important point in choosing your expedition leader. Choose him carefully, very carefully indeed.

I have followed in his footsteps in Southern Morocco and climbed the High Atlas Mountains and trudged in the sands of the northern Sahara Desert. I have plodded wearily in the Northern Frontier District of Kenya in the Huri Hills and undergone a near fatal trip with him crossing the Chalbi Desert. I have also followed him into Zimbabwe and Botswana, in the Okavango Delta and Kalahari Desert.

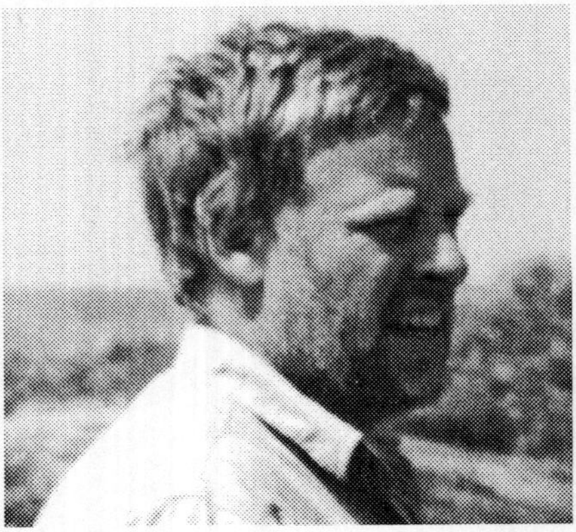

PETER DRAKE
The friend whose footsteps I followed.
This photograph was taken in the Matopos Hills, Zimbabwe

I have been hungry and thirsty. I have lived on baked beans, pilchards and corned beef for weeks on end. I have been filthy and smelly and not had the luxury of a wash for up to two weeks. I have felt exhausted and tired, frightened and intimidated, lonely and depressed, but I have never regretted one single moment of it.

If medical expeditions interest you then my advice is

to follow your instincts and go. Do not expect it to be easy because it will not be, but the rewards and experiences will be beyond your wildest dreams.

The purpose of the book is to give you some idea of the places I have travelled to but more especially to give an account of the people I have met in my capacity as a doctor. As well as travelling in northern, eastern and southern Africa I spent two weeks in China working in a hospital in Beijing studying the ancient art of acupuncture. I have met nurses and doctors in these areas and have treated people myself in these often remote areas. Many people have left an indelible memory.

At the end of the book is an account of my experiences with snakes and, on a more serious note, how to deal with the more common emergencies you may come across on expeditions and when using travel medicine.

When I returned home I would bore the girls at work with my exploits and they would listen patiently and carefully. In retrospect I must have bored them to death! One day Elizabeth suggested that I write them all down in the form of a book as I suspect they would rather read about them instead of having to listen! I had never thought of it until it was mentioned and over the years have collected stories of my adventures. Jane and Wendy helped me to start it off but it was the original suggestion by Elizabeth that started the ball rolling. I am grateful to them all.

MOROCCO

TELOUET, WILD LAVENDER AND SHOOTING STARS

Morocco is situated at the north end of Africa and borders both the Atlantic Ocean and the Mediterranean Sea. It also has land borders with Algeria and the Sahara Desert. It has some 1,500 miles of coastline and several mountain ranges.

During the twelfth century BC Phoenician traders established commercial posts on both its Mediterranean and North Atlantic coast and when Carthage fell to Rome in 146BC Roman influence and trade expanded into northern Morocco, but the country was left under the rule of its own Berber kings. Direct Roman rule was later established in 19AD when the Roman Emperor had the Berber king murdered. Roman influence was already strong and quickly spreading and it can still be seen today at various excavation sites, notably the ruins of Volubilis near Meknes. Later, as Christianity spread, evidence emerged that the Berbers too may have become Christianised.

Before Rome fell in the fifth century AD the Roman administration of Morocco had virtually ceased and Huns, Vandals and Visigoths raided the region without actually settling there. In the seventh century AD the first wave of westward Arab expansion reached Morocco and for the following two centuries, despite many Berber revolts, the Arabs held on, the country remained strong and the influence of Islam was consolidated.

The end of the eighth century saw the establishment of Morocco's first ruling dynasty and a centralised government was started by Moulay Idress l. His son Moulay Idress ll founded Fez as his capital in 808AD but, after his death, the kingdom split up and a Berber Confederation for a time governed the lands.

In the eleventh century Youssef ben Tachfine, leader of the veiled fanatical tribe of nomad Berbers from the Sahara, began his conquest of Morocco and in 1062 Marrakesh was founded. By the time Youssef ben Tachfine died in 1106 his power had extended into Europe. This dynasty was eventually overthrown by another confederation of Berber tribes, this time from the High Atlas, who conquered Marrakesh in 1147. Some of the

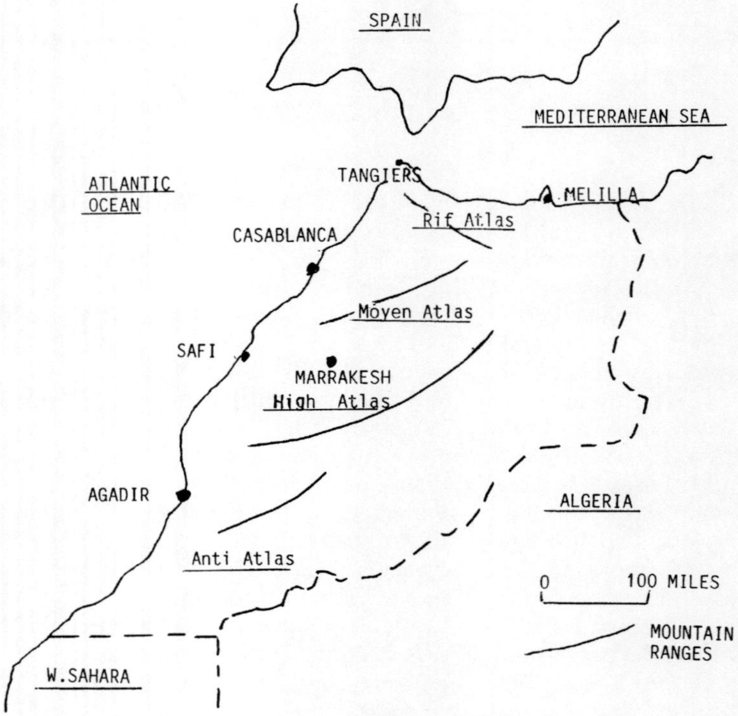

MOROCCO AND THE ATLAS MOUNTAINS

finest Hispano-Moorish architecture to be seen in the country can be accredited to this dynasty. This dynasty in turn began to crumble and eventually collapsed in 1492 when yet another nomadic Berber tribe from Eastern Morocco came to power . After two centuries their power also faded.

During this time the Portuguese set up settlements at various points along the coast and the country was again united by Saadians from the Zagora region in the Draa Valley against both the Portuguese and the Spaniards. They ruled successfully for about a century and during this time established better relations with their European neighbours.

The Saadians in their turn were displaced by another family from the Hedjaz, the Alaouites, who made themselves powerful in the Tafilalet and still rule Morocco today.

The outstanding figure in this dynasty was Sultan Moulay Ismail who lived from 1672-1727 and he drove out all the foreign

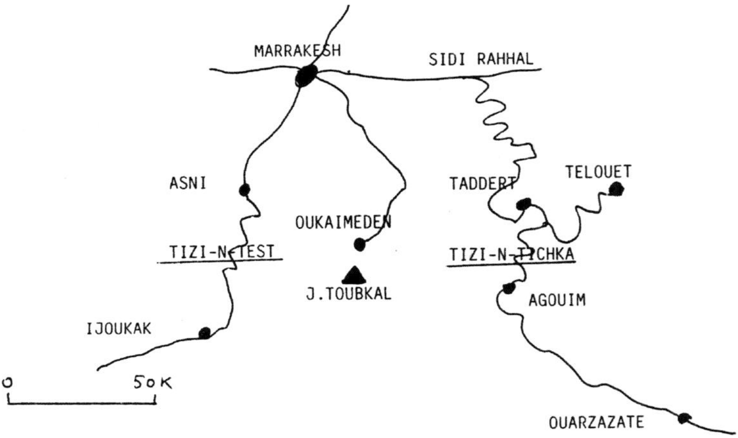

WEST HIGH ATLAS

nationals from Morocco except for the towns of Ceuta and Melilla, both of which remained in Spanish hands.

In the nineteenth and twentieth centuries Morocco began to disintegrate, partly through increasing contact with European power and partly through internal rivalries.

In 1912 France and Spain, with the approval of Britain and Germany, divided all Morocco except Tangiers which became an international zone. The arrangement took the form of a protectorate with the Sultan remaining the country's ruler, but having no real power. Morocco, however, was not fully pacified by the French until 1934 and even then there were zones of dissidence, especially to the south and in the High Atlas. The most notorious group of Berbers who resisted French domination lived and ruled from the kasbah at Telouet. This was the home of the Lords of the Atlas and it was there that we visited on our return trip to Marrakesh after a visit to the sand sea in the northern Sahara Desert.

The trip from a medical point of view had been a nightmare. High temperatures travelling in vehicles across the desert coupled with an outbreak of gastroenteritis had kept me very busy. Within the space of a few hours members of the expedition were dropping like flies - dehydrated, toxic and very ill. As we once again ascended the Tizi-n-Tichka Pass the temperature dropped noticeably and the health of the expedition as a whole started to improve. We camped on the side of the track that led down to the village of Telouet. I once again drew breath and tried to sort the expedition out before we proceeded the next day to the village. We arrived about lunch time and I can remember feeling disappointed as we drew into the centre of the square. It could best be described as a one-horse town. The stone buildings crowded around the square and the whole place gave an impression of being untidy and unkempt. However, the main reason for our visit was to see the kasbah at Telouet. We camped about two miles from the village in a stony area where wild lavender grew.

Soon after we had set up camp Peter vanished into the village and later returned saying that he had organised a guide to show us around the castle. I do not know how he did it, I did not ask, I just accepted it. Peter Drake is a genius at organisation and this was another example. Those who were fit set off to visit the fabled kasbah. The first appearance was majestic and as we approached we realised how enormous it was. There were storks nesting on the battlements while vultures circled overhead. The kasbah stands at some 8,000 feet in the High Atlas and, apart from occasional small trees and shrubs, the scene is dominated by rocks and mountains.

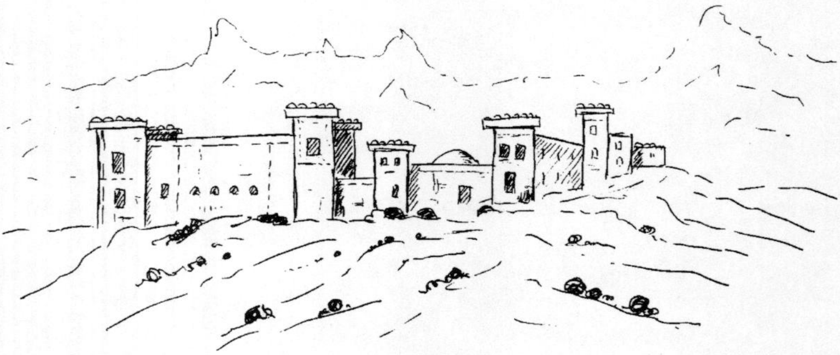

MOROCCAN KASBAH OR CASTLE AT TELOUET

It was here that local people could seek refuge when under threat from attack. Trade centres were formed here usually inside the castle walls and they became the nucleus of towns and later cities. Marrakesh is a good example of this.

The history of the kasbah at Telouet is a monument to cruelty and barbarism. The fanatical tribe of Berbers who dominated the region were the Glaoui and slaughtered and killed anyone who dared to defy them. They accumulated great wealth not only be their piratical activities but also from the salt mines they owned. These were visited by caravans from the Sahara and from the Sudan. The Glaoui not only raised the price of salt but also demanded taxes from the camel caravans. To discover more about the barbarism and mediaeval ways of the Glaoui I suggest you read The Lords of the Atlas by Gavin Maxwell. It will fire your imagination and curdle your blood.

We approached the main gates, some twenty feet in height, by a ramp which led from the path. The guide struggled with a huge bunch of keys and eventually, after creaking and groaning, the enormous doors opened. We found ourselves in a square with the ground sloping to the left covered in black beetles. It was difficult to place our feet on the floor without crushing them. As I looked up there were wooden balconies overlooking the square in various stages of neglect. Behind were the remains of what I presumed had been the stables. To the left of the square was a small doorway which led to a twisting and narrow stone staircase. We followed the guide slowly upwards and found ourselves at the end of a long corridor at the far end of which were another pair of huge wooden doors. He once again struggled with his keys and what then enfolded belonged to another world. The decor was magnificent despite the years of neglect. The floor was of stone and marble; the walls were covered in tiles and huge columns supported the wooden roof which was carved and painted. There was ample evidence of beautifully worked plaster. The whole appearance was a mixture of Italian, Spanish and Moroccan workmanship and no expense had been spared. No wonder it was referred to as the Palace of a Thousand and one Nights. I was brought back to earth however, by standing in some bat droppings in the corner of the room! This was one of those occasions when you had to pinch yourself to make sure you were there.

We left the room and after the guide had once again locked the doors I discovered the handles and bolts were made of silver. We then ascended another twisting staircase and walked onto a roof space. The views overlooking the surrounding mountains were magnificent. The roof tiles were green - a mark of importance. I slipped one into my trousers feeling a little guilty, but I did it anyway. After about half an hour we left the kasbah and headed back to the camp site. Here I confessed my crime to Peter and broke the tile in half and gave him one half. He smiled at me and put it into his rucksack. I learned later he had broken his tile in half and given it to a friend!

We returned to the camp site amongst the wild lavender and, after a hot meal, settled down for the night. I was awoken during the night to attend to yet another member of the party who had fallen to the outbreak of dysentery. By this time I was running very short of medical supplies and was beginning to get concerned about the health of the expedition as a whole. I returned to my camp bed amidst the glorious smell of the wild lavender and what had been a day of many emotions was capped by watching shooting stars against the star-studded black African night.

In 1956 Morocco became totally independent after years of violence and repression. The government since that time has done much to lift the standards of the country. Today Morocco is a stable country and ruled over by their King, King Hassan ll who ascended the throne in February 1961 on the death of his father.

Geographically the country can be divided into four basic types. There is a western plain but mountains form a large part of the country. In the north are the Rif Atlas and the Middle Atlas, but extending for hundreds of miles in an east-westerly direction are the High Atlas Mountains. These lie some fifty miles south of Marrakesh and are crossed by Tizi-n-Tichka Pass in the east and the Tizi-n-Test Pass in the west. These cut off the highest mountains which form the Central Massif. The highest mountain here is Jbel Toubkal and it is to here that we were heading, which is at some 13,700 feet. There is a sub-Sahara region which begins in the southern slopes of the High Atlas and descends through the foothills and subsidiary ranges to the sand desert a hundred to a hundred and twenty miles away. On the eastern side of the country is a stony high plateau region.

The indigenous population is largely Arabic and the influence of Islam is considerable. They range from sedentary farmers in the north to nomadic herders in the south. The principal tribe is the Berbers though there are pockets of Jews and other non-indigenous people to be found, but these are mainly in the north.

The religion of Morocco is mainly Moslem and this is appreciated as in the morning you are often woken by the people being called to prayer. There are, however, people of both Catholic and Jewish religions.

In some parts of Morocco the women still cover their faces with a veil and photography should be carried out with discretion. I have known members of an expedition trying to take photographs of women only to receive a volley of several rocks heading in their direction! It is important also when in remote or holy places that a camera should only be used with discretion. If you ask politely local people will allow you to take their photographs, but they usually expect something in return.

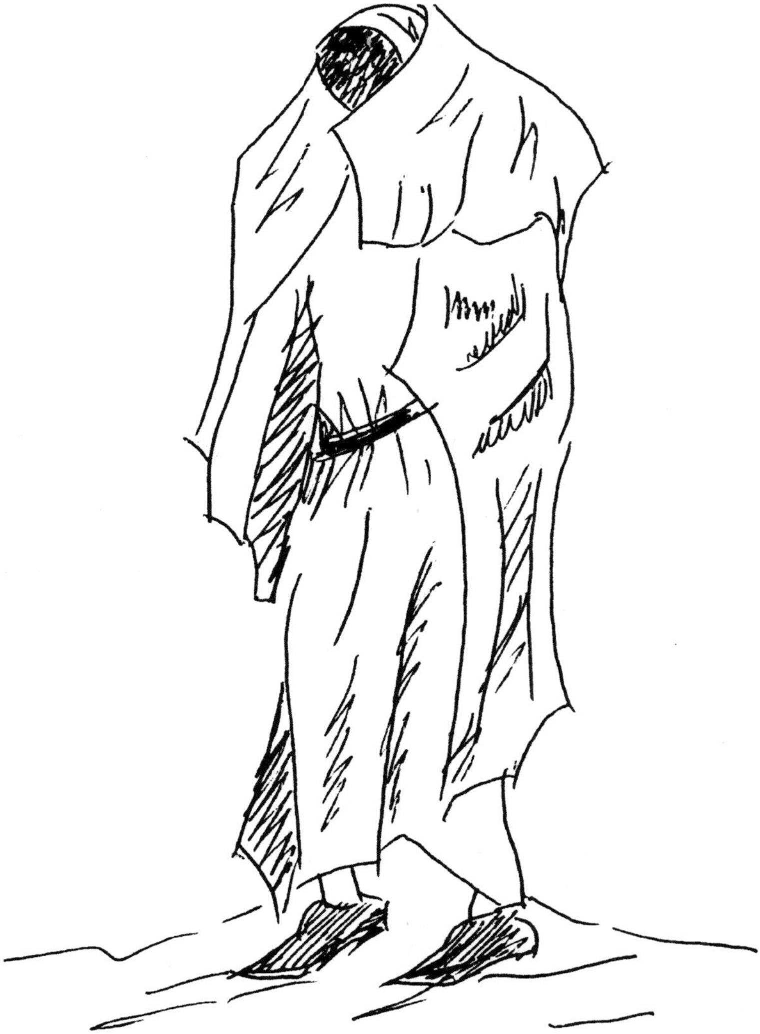

MOROCCAN WOMAN

THE BERBERS

The people of Morocco can be divided roughly into the urban and rural populations. The Berbers who are the indigenous race are still more likely to live in the mountains and countryside. They migrated here in the face of the Arab invaders from the east and they have tended to settle in the towns and cities. The Berbers are of three main types. The Rifians inhabit the north, the Chleuhs are from the Middle and High Atlas and the Siussi are found mainly in the southwest. The origin of the Berbers is not known with certainty but they are thought to have originated in Europe. Today most Moroccans are of mixed race and it is difficult to say if one is pure Berber or Arabic or Black African. However, there are areas in Erfoud and in the Draa Valley where Berber blood is virtually pure. There Berbers have a different language to the Arab but they can usually understand Arabic. The reverse is not true.

Throughout time Morocco has been invaded and influenced by external forces. The Romans, the Arabs and the Europeans, and their intrusion has been fiercely resisted. The Berbers were keen and able fighting men and at one time their influence extended into Spain, and even when they were not fighting against outsiders they fought amongst themselves for control. However, today the Berbers live a relatively simple life. They have become the farmers and shepherds, quite a change from their aggressive predecessors. They have little in the way of possessions and live in close-knit communities. They tend their goats, sheep and cattle and own farms growing maize and other crops. In the High Atlas there is a mixture of Arab and Berber blood and it is the call to Allah that wakens you in the mountain villages like Imlil - certainly a pleasant change from your alarm clock! In the more remote villages like Sidi Chamharouch, the influence of Islam fades and the Berbers have their own religion. Sidi Chamharouch is a holy village to the Barbers and they appear to be very secretive about it. When we visited Sidi Chamharouch to see its holy temple with its white-painted roof adorned with flags nobody ventured anywhere near it and when questions were asked no answers were forthcoming. We were left in no doubt about their feelings and certainly no photographs were taken.

It appeared strange to me that such a proud and noble tribe now lived such a simple way of life in the mountains. I am in no doubt about their abilitity to control their future and the way they now exist only endeared them to me. They are a very caring community. We witnessed the whole family from grandparents to children living under one roof. They were very keen to seek medical help, once they knew of our presence, for any member of the family who was ill. They seemed to be entirely self-sufficient and relied on no one for their needs. The principles by which they lived are to be admired. They were generous to others, polite and courteous and cheerful and well mannered. They were not against making a quick profit, but who is not. They had little in the way of wealth and exhibited many of the qualities which we could do well to copy. It struck me that two different religions can exist in relative harmony side by side without bloodshed or marked aggression. If only this could be copied in other parts of the world!

The pastures they had in the mountains we visited were sparse indeed and the shepherds led their goats and sheep up and down the valleys in search of grazing land yet they seemed to survive despite the rugged conditions. They obtained milk from their goats and wool from the sheep and the more prosperous

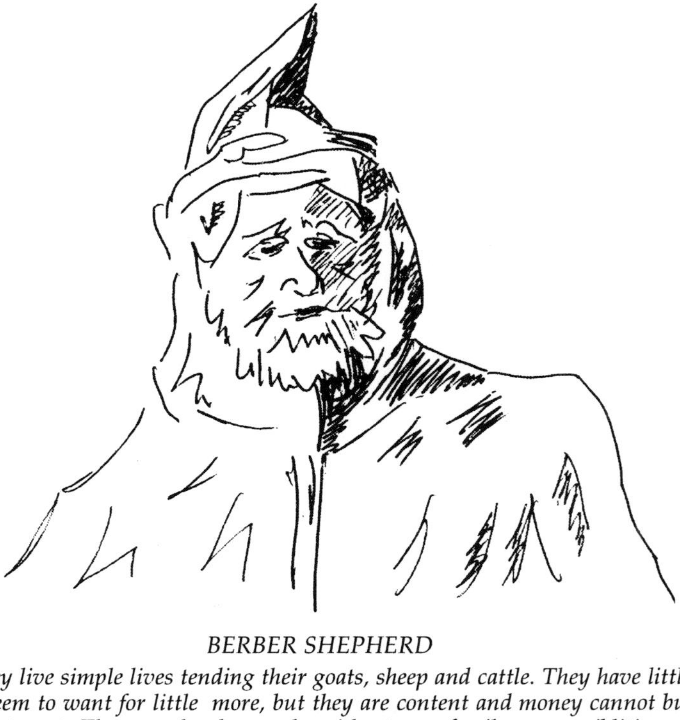

BERBER SHEPHERD

They live simple lives tending their goats, sheep and cattle. They have little, and seem to want for little more, but they are content and money cannot buy contentment. They are hardy people with strong family responsiblities, all members living under one roof from children to grand-parents. Their homes are often shared with their cattle and chickens. They are a proud mountain people commanding respect and admiration, living in harsh conditions.

obtained dairy products from their cattle. Chickens were also a familiar site in homes we visited. The farmers grew maize and other crops and had developed an ingenious system of irrigation. They were certainly masters at this.

Conditions in the summer when we visited were favourable to their way of life but winter must have posed a different problem. The temperature even in the summer fell to below freezing at night and there was still snow in the mountain gullies. All of the summer must be geared to surviving the harsh winter: storing and collecting of food and fuel for survival. We discovered in Imlil that the more wealthy move to more temperate climates when winter approaches.

The clothing worn by the Berbers in the mountains varied enormously. The older people tended to wear the more traditional dress. Men had turbans on their heads and wore long heavy woollen djellabahs or kaftans with sandals on their feet. The women and young girls wore kaftans which were lighter and more brightly coloured and adorned with heavy Berber jewellery. The younger men and boys had migrated to a more European form of dress with sweaters, trousers and trainers. A popular form of footwear in the mountains was nicknamed Michelin wellies by the expedition members and these took the form of discarded car tyres cut up to form sandals. These were ideal for the mountain way of life and the Berbers could leap from rock to rock in relative safety.

We took dehydrated food with us and lived mainly on this but we did have the opportunity to sample the local dishes. In Imlil rice, lamb and chickens were available, as well as locally made bread. The meats were often served as a kebab but lamb was also served as tajine. This is a lamb stew with added vegetables. Couscous is a rice dish accompanied by chicken and vegetables and this also proved to be popular. The bread was served round and flat but soon became stale and inedible. Alcohol was available, although not in the mountains, in the form of beer and wine. The beer is brewed locally and the best known wines come from the areas of Fez and Meknes. The most common local drink we enjoyed in the mountains was mint tea. The mint leaves were placed either in the teapot or in the glasses in which the tea was served. These were small and round and the tea was served hot and sweet. The custom of drinking mint tea was often used as a greeting of friendship or a way of saying thank you.

Morocco is a stable country and retains many of its traditional ways. It has been influenced by western ideas but the balance has been successfully managed. The Moroccans are keen to seek help and form ties with western culture and yet the balance they have to maintain with their neighbours must be difficult.

MARRAKESH

On my first visit to Morocco we stayed at the camp site near the centre of Marrakesh, but on my second visit we stayed at a School for the Blind. The arrangement Peter had made with the principal was that we could use the facilities of the school providing we painted some of the classrooms. The agreement worked very well. We had the use of the kitchens, dining room and showers and, more importantly a secure place to leave some of our equipment not needed on the trip. The blind school was in easy reach of the centre of Marrakesh.

Marrakesh is one of the jewels of Morocco and a variety of different styles of architecture can be found. The city gardens are well cared for and attended but, for the traveller, the Arab market, or souk, holds the greatest interest and attraction. Like many other cities Marrakesh grew around a fortified settlement where local people could seek refuge when under threat of attack. Markets were soon established inside and it became a centre for trade and consequently grew and expanded. The original settlement is still there with a large square in front of it in the famous Djemaa el Fna. This became a gathering place for merchants, touts, beggars, water-sellers, acrobats, snake-charmers, medicine men and performers of each and every sort. The original walls can still be entered by various gateways. Also in the square are stalls selling various goods, open-air cafes and most exotic stalls selling spices. The smells that abound are fantastic. Pickpockets also abound, we found to our cost, so beware! A good vantage point to overlook the square is the Cafe de France where you can drink beer and soak up the atmosphere.

Inside the souk lies a different world but you really need a guide to show you around. There are no shortage of willing volunteers but at a price! There is a maze of narrow streets and markets and the latter tend to be grouped together depending on what they are selling. There are copper smiths, jewellers, traders in leather, woollen goods and carpets and craftsmen working in wood. The place and atmosphere is absolutely magical although it may appear a little daunting at first. Again I kept pinching myself to make sure I was actually there. Trading is by the barter system and it is prudent to try and obtain your purchase for about a third of the price they are asking. If they are unwilling to

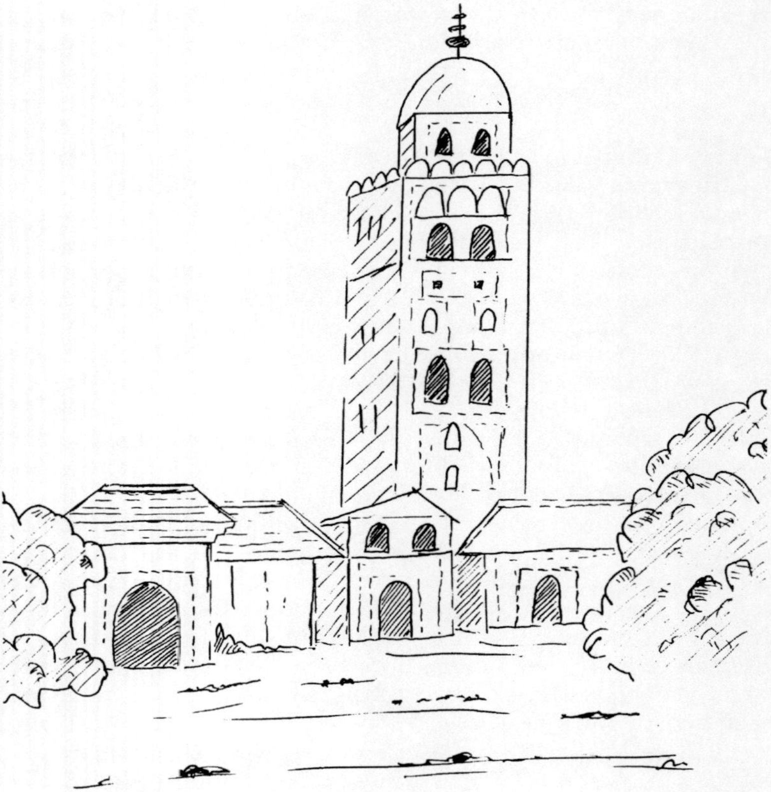

KOUTOUBIA MOSQUE IN MARRAKESH

It is the highest building in the city. Building started in about 1150 and took some 40 years to complete. It is some 50 metres high and regarded as being the symbol of Marrakesh. It also served as a model for other mosques built in Morocco and similar buildings can be found in Spain when Moroccan influence spread there.

sell, go somewhere else and up the price a little. This will be about the right price you should pay.

Marrakesh is a city full of contrast and is divided into the Arab and French European parts. Most of the interest, however, lies in the Arab quarter. The High Atlas Mountains form a spectacular backdrop some fifty miles south and it was to here that we were travelling next.

THE HIGH ATLAS MOUNTAINS

The Atlas Mountains extend a total of 1,200 miles from Tunisia in the east to the western part of Morocco and comprise six groups; the first four lie in Morocco and the last two extend into part of the Algeria. The peaks of the Anti and Middle Atlas reach over 11,000 feet, but for the mountaineer the High Atlas remain the most important group. This area was first visited by Charles de Foucauld in about 1883. Even today little climbing has been done outside the Toubkal Massif. The French who occupied Morocco early this century were the chief pioneers. The French Alpine Club were responsible for building The Neltner Hut at the base of Mount Toubkal. This was built as a mountaineering hut but is also used as a ski shelter. Both rock-climbing and skiing were enjoyed by the French in the mountains but both of these activities have declined since Morocco became independent and the French withdrew. The Neltner Hut was built in 1938 and is a stone-built, two-storey mountain refuge hut. It has a substantial roof and adjacent outbuildings. It stands at some 10,500 feet and is the highest refuge hut in the range. The ground floor consists of a common room and kitchen where gas stoves are provided. Upstairs is a dormitory consisting of alpine-style bunk beds able to sleep some twenty people. A rescue stretcher is kept in the hut and there is a guardian who is responsible for the maintenance and running of the hut. He could often be seen burning rubbish at the back of the hut and generally keeping it spick and span.

The best seasons to climb these magnificent mountains are the spring and autumn, but for the serious winter climber the High Atlas also offer great possibilities. In spring snow and rock climbing alternate, while in September the peaks are dry and travel on foot is easy. The rock is variable and usually best along the ridges. We felt that rock climbing would be dangerous as the rock seemed friable, presumably being exposed to a wide range of climatic conditions. It was something I would not have contemplated: I had enough problems walking along the ridges! The highest mountain in the range is Toubkal at 13,700 feet and is the peak most mountaineers head for, but it is by no means the most beautiful. One member on my first ascent described it as climbing a great slag heap! Such is the reward for taking a young explorer to northern Africa to climb mountains!

Apart from climbing, the traveller in the High Atlas cannot help being charmed by the valley terraces of maize, the ingenious irrigation systems, the ochre and red hillsides and the varying vegetation on the richer northern slopes and the arid Saharan landscape. He will enjoy meeting the Berbers who wrestle hard in the harsh mountain environment. Bird life and insect life abound, especially the butterflies. There were even butterflies near the summit of Toubkal!

On my first trip to Morocco in 1975 we left Heathrow airport and some 2,500 miles later found ourselves in Marrakesh landing in the evening. We camped overnight and fifty miles later, south of Marrakesh, we arrived in the High Atlas. We walked and climbed our way to the Neltner Hut and all this we achieved in just over twenty-four hours! I must have been mad at the time.

Any information about the High Atlas was sketchy at the time and not very informative. We left in some fear and trepidation but the conditions we met were not very different from situations you may find in the British Isles. The main difference was the variation in temperature certainly hotter during the day and at night it froze. The technical difficulties were no different from some of the ridge walking in Scotland due to the friability of the rock but providing you did not venture too close to the edge you were in little danger.

The flight from Heathrow via Lisbon and Tangiers took about four hours travelling with Air Maroc. We travelled in considerable comfort and the meals on board were excellent. It was a good way to start a mountaineering expedition and one I can recommend. Within hours of our arrival we had reached our base camp in Marrakesh. The camp site was crowded with many campers, there was a small shop and doubtful toilet facilities. This was borne out by the graffiti on the toilet walls. The one that made me laugh the most was 'this shit house is really a shit house!' It certainly lived up to that reputation. After a night's sleep we left the following morning heading south towards Asni on the Tizi-n-Test Pass, one of the passes that crosses the High Atlas. I remember before we left the camp site a French tourist in his super desert vehicle, which ran on both petrol and diesel, pressed the wrong switch and flooded the petrol part of his engine with diesel. I could not help but laugh as he cursed his misfortune. He was certainly not a happy man! How much more simple life is for the locals who travel perched on the backs of their donkeys with a smile on their faces. I thought the comparison was highly amusing at the time!

The road heading south from Marrakesh was long and straight before it began to turn and twist as it approached the foothills of the mountains. The road was well tarmacked, but as far as we were concerned when it reached Asni that was the end of comfortable travelling. Asni is a small Berber community on the pass. There are stone-built houses by the roadside and several small stalls selling rock specimens and geodes. The children crowded around us trying to sell us their samples of rocks but seemed content with the sweets and biscuits which they received in return.

The main reason for travelling to Asni was to turn off the main road and make our way to Imlil where the next phase of the expedition would begin. However, just through Asni on the left-hand side of the road is the Hotel Toubkal and this was another reason for stopping there. The hotel is of high Moroccan standard with sufficient parking facilities at the front. Inside, it is beautifully decorated and there is an ample supply of good food and wine and a comfortable bed for the night. The gardens in the rear are well tended and cared for and look onto the stunning scene of the snow-capped High Atlas Mountains in the distance. The other great asset the hotel has is a swimming pool which, as you can imagine, was very popular with the members of the expedition.

The dirt road that leads from Asni to Imlil is about five miles and twists and turns through the valleys and opens up onto spectacular views of the mountains. There are steep cliffs on one side of the road and sudden deep drops on the other. This became a familiar scene in our travels in the High Atlas, whether in a vehicle, sitting on a mule or just walking.

We arrived at Imlil some hours later after negotiating areas of the road which had been washed away by the rainfall in the winter and it was our intention to spend the night there. The Berber village of Imlil comprises a number of single and two-storey stone buildings with the main approach road ending at a car park in front of a small hotel. We were immediately approached by the local muleteers and guides and in a small cafe negotiated a deal for the mules to take us to the Neltner hut. This was a distance of some eight miles and a climb of some five thousand feet. It was our original plan to spend the night here, but we were assured that mules could be arranged immediately and so we left the same afternoon. We hired ten mules together with the muleteers and agreed to pay them when they had delivered us to our destination. The gear was loaded onto the mules in wicker panniers and we set off on foot following behind. Before we left we were asked to sign a book so that they could record our departure into the mountains. We also found out pretty quickly that the charge for this was one dirham each, so we decided not to bother!

The path twists and turns and winds its way out of Imlil and onto the Plain of Arond through fields of maize and walnut groves. As you leave Imlil at the far end of the village you pass more houses and a few shops crowded along the side of the track. There were shops selling meat and a general store. We also passed the local hairdresser cutting his clients' hair whilst sitting under a tree and the area where the mules were kept under the shade of walnut trees. Once on the plain you find yourself amongst the most spectacular mountain scenery. On the hills surrounding you are further Berber settlements, stone-built with flat roofs huddled together and clinging to the sides of the steep mountain slopes. The children from the villages were eager to come and see us pass, dressed in their traditional costumes. They were after anything they could get, usually sweets and cigarettes. The whole place and its atmosphere was magical. The march from Imlil proceeded at a brisk pace and it was not long before the party split into two groups. Needless to say I helped to bring up the rear in the second. The route from Imlil to Sidi Chamharouch, which was our next port of call, followed the river up into the mountains.

EVENTS THAT UNFOLDED IN THE ATLAS MOUNTAINS

It was a dull and overcast day and some members had decided to cook inside their tents. I was reading in our tent, only to be jolted into activity by a loud explosion in the adjoining tent. I thought it had been struck by lightning. I dashed outside to find the tent in flames and a young scout rushing up the track towards the Neltner hut screaming in pain and holding his face in his hands. In true and gallant fashion I ran after him, caught him up, to find him in tears and almost hysterical. I comforted him by putting my arms around him and then took a pace back. His face was red and extensively burned, his eyebrows and lashes had disappeared, and his hair and sweater badly singed. I brought him back to the camp site, put him in someone else's sleeping bag and sedated him to calm him down and relieve his pain. I organised a nurse to sit with him and comfort him and kept him under observation for the rest of the day. The other members organised a rota system to stay with him and he spent the rest of the day sleeping. By the next day he had sufficiently recovered to continue his so-called expedition. It turned out that whilst cooking in his tent the gas supply had run out and inside the tent he had changed gas cylinders and the residual gas escaped. He then lit the new gas supply and the result was there for all to see. He would not be going that again in a hurry! We

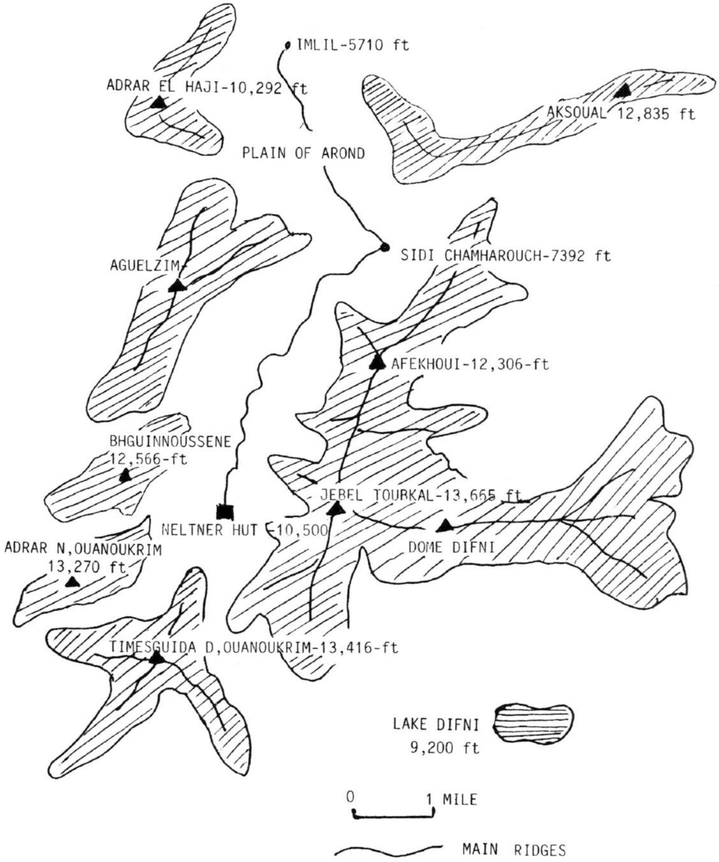

THE JOURNEY FROM IMLIL TO THE NELTNER HUT

spent the evening preparing for our assault of Toubkal accompanied by a supply of alcohol!

We woke early the next day at about six o'clock and after several hot drinks started our ascent. It was at this time that one of the girls in the party started to hyperventilate. Her breathing became faster and faster and she ended up in tears. I calmed her down and comforted her and she soon recovered. Needless to say, she spent the rest of the day in camp, but much to her credit she climbed the mountain two days later. Hyper-ventilation is a common problem on expeditions and for any aspiring expedition doctors it is important to carry a paper bag in your back pocket!

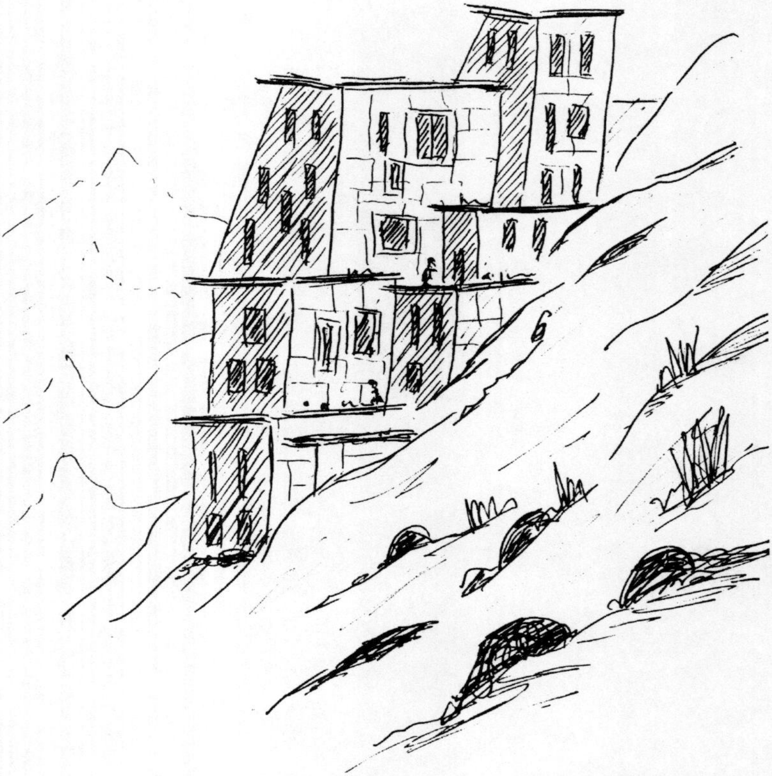

BERBER VILLAGE CLINGING TO STEEP MOUNTAIN SIDE

On leaving the camp we commenced our ascent by crossing the stream onto a scree field on the left-hand side of the valley. By keeping to the left-hand side amongst larger boulders we made fairly rapid progress until we reached an upper valley below the final ridge. By this time the sun had risen and the temperature rose rapidly. By ascending the right-hand side of the upper valley we eventually reached the ridge that would lead us to the summit. The ridge had precipitate drops to the right-hand side and about eleven o'clock we reached the summit. The views were magnificent, we could see the foothills that led south to the Sahara Desert and to the north was the area that we had walked in from two days before. At the summit is a huge steel erection which was a popular place to have your photograph taken. Most of the members were fit and well but a few had headaches and felt a little sick. After a rest and a drink we slowly started our descent. We came down the valley to the north of the summit and enjoyed some fabulous scree runs. In this valley we found the wreck of an aeroplane which had crashed some five years before. It was definitely an eerie and disturbing experience. I expected to hear people crying for help but there was only a stony silence. We finally returned to base camp at about three o'clock, all safe and sound.

The evenings were magical. We sat and talked after our meal, and sang-songs around the fire and the spirit of the expedition was high. The shepherds passed up and down the valley each day setting off in the morning to return at night with their goats and sheep. The sounds they made and the ringing of the bells around some of the animals necks would echo in the valley between the mountains. It really was a most enchanting place and the memories have lasted for many years. The Neltner hut was a popular place for the Berber shepherds to meet and camp at night. They would sit by their fires and drink mint tea and on occasions would come to our camp site. They communicated to us in broken French and conversation was difficult. They usually wanted cigarettes, matches or sweets but they were able to give us in exchange valuable information about paths and routes in the mountains. They often benefited from medical help and were always grateful for it. These hill shepherds were extremely poor and would regularly sift through our rubbish tip looking for polythene bags and whatever they could use. I remember the remains of the burnt tent disappearing rapidly!

In the High Atlas mountains is Lake Difni which is visited regularly by the Berbers who regard it as a holy place. They way to the lake is approached by heading up the far end of the valley beyond the Neltner Hut and climbing a col into the next valley. The lake is a considerable journey into this valley and several hours march. It was to here that we next decided to go. We were late setting off and reached the col by late morning. It was apparent to me that there was no way the journey could be accomplished that day and a much earlier start was needed. I made my feelings known and suggested we returned to camp. The leader decided to go on and I volunteered to take anyone who did not wish to go back. The other party of eight decided to continue so I and the others wandered slowly back admiring the magnificent scenery. At camp we had a lazy day sorting our gear out and generally tidying the camp. After our evening meal we sat and talked and as darkness started to fall three of us went up to the far end of the valley to await the return of the other group.

We returned after about an hour having taken torches and whistles with us. We had returned empty handed - there was no sign of them. At first light the next day I organised two groups, one to go and stay on the col and the other to walk to the far end of the valley. All the time we kept in visual contact of each other. It struck me as amusing at the time the idea of not losing a search party in search of another group that had become lost. I made sure that did not happen! By late morning they appeared at the far end of the valley, tired, bedraggled and obviously very glad to see us again. Fortunately nobody had come to any harm but some of the members had obviously been frightened by their ordeal. They had lost their way and spent the night sheltering in a cave. I had a few quiet words with the leader and I am afraid to say our relationship took a rapid nose-dive. There is no excuse for foolhardy behaviour in the mountains, not only does it put the leader's life at risk it also jeopardises the safety of younger members. It would be far better if such individuals stayed at home and common sense could prevail.

The following day I returned to Marrakesh and another doctor replaced me in the mountains. I had enjoyed most of my time there despite the problems I had encountered.

ALI-BEN-BRAHEIM

My second visit to the High Atlas was in 1988; my first being in 1975. As I approached Sidi Chamharouch all those years ago I was tired and weary trying to keep up with the mules. Teenagers of the village rushed out to sell us bottles of orange and Coca Cola which they had kept cool in buckets of water taken from the river. I bought a drink, sat on a rock and tried to catch my breath and quench my not inconsiderable thirst. Most of the village had turned out to see the mule train plodding its weary way on and up into the mountains. Before I left I decided that another drink was in order and bought one from another of the youngsters keen to sell them to us. As I started to drink it there was a yell and a shout behind me and I turned round to see the young lad who had sold me the drink lying on the floor. Blood was coming from his head and another pool was rapidly forming by his outstretched hand. The first young Berber that had sold me the drink had attacked the second, smashing his head, and, as he had put up his hand to protect himself, had severed his radial artery and gashed his head with a bottle. This was big trouble. The villagers gathered round him and me, as I was by now bending over him trying to comfort him and find out exactly what

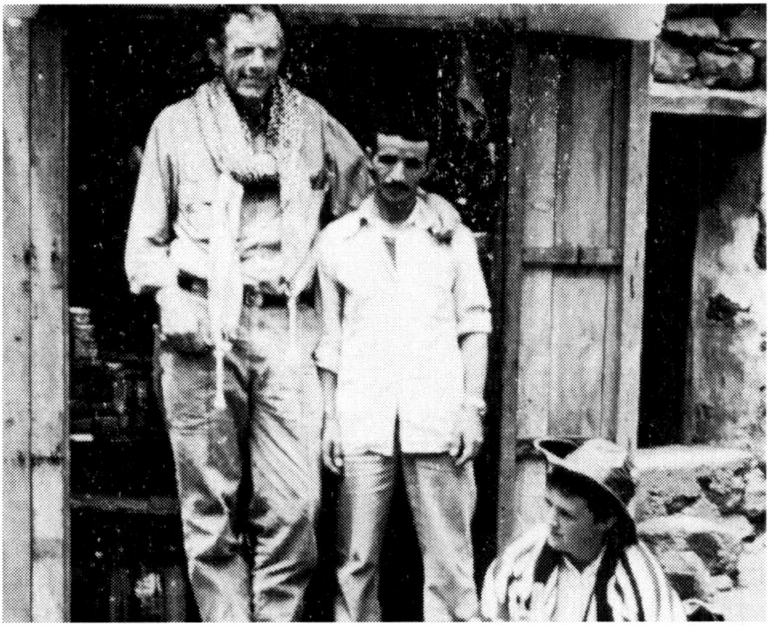

ALI BEN BRAHEIM

He lives with his wife and family in Siddi Chamharouch. He owns a small shop selling prayer beads, tins of food and clothing. A small man, courteous and blessed with a sense of humour. When showing gratitude he shakes your hand for what seems ages, his whole body becomes involved. He supplements his income by helping expeditions venturing into the mountains with the help of his mule – Sirdun. I will never forget my encounters with this loveable man.

had happened. Fortunately, an elder of the village was there and as I talked to him he managed to calm everybody down. I took off my belt and tore my shirt up, dressed and stopped the bleeding artery and urgently sent for the medical gear which by this time had left the village on the back of a mule and had gone further up into the mountains towards the Neltner Hut. I think it was then that the villagers realised we were trying to help the unfortunate lad and the atmosphere which had been very tense seemed to settle down. I spoke to the elder and told him as best I could that we would take the young lad with us, dress his wounds and return him later. As I look back on that incident I sometimes shudder when I think what may have happened. I think at first they thought we were trying to kidnap him but they eventually agreed to let him go and we led the unfortunate victim, sitting on a mule, out of the village to await the arrival of the medical equipment.

About half an hour later a member of the expedition came running down the path with my medical bag, having received our urgent message. He was totally and utterly exhausted and the first thing we had to do was to revive him. We then lifted the young boy off his mule and sat him on a rock by the side of the path. Ten minutes later, and with three stitches in a head wound and several more in his wrist, a great smile appeared on his face and he started jumping around with great glee and delight. We instantly became good friends. As I was bandaging his wounds three young boys from the village were seen running up the path towards us from Sidi Chamharouch carrying a tray of mint tea. We recognised this as a way of saying thank you so we sat by the side of the path drinking the tea and catching our breath once again.

The young boy was called Ali ben Braheim and the poor boy thought he had finished with doctors for the day, but his wounds were both deep and he needed penicillin by injection to make sure they did not become infected. Trying to explain this to him was not easy and he was obviously not keen on the idea when he realised where I was going to put my needle! He shot off up the path at great speed. I ran after him, rugby-tackled him and before he knew it I injected my penicillin into his buttocks. We were soon rolling on the floor, laughing and giggling and he looked at me with a smile on his face. I was amazed. Penicillin injections can be very painful. We both then stood up and he began to shake me vigorously by the hand. We returned to the place we had drunk the mint tea and his fellow villagers looked at us in astonishment. After a short time and a discussion with him and his friends I allowed him to return to his village but insisted that I saw him the next day . We then once again set off for the Neltner hut which was still two hours' away. Once again I was glad to see my bed!

The next day, as I was sorting my gear out outside my tent, striding up the path came Ali ben Braheim with his mule called Sirdun. We sat down and started chatting as best we could and I made him some tea and gave him biscuits. He had come to say thank you and show me his wounds. My work the previous day was satisfactory and there had been no more bleeding. I once again dressed his wounds and asked to see him again in a couple of days. After about half an hour he once again left in the direction of his village after another vigorous session of shaking hands!

On my first visit I stayed in the mountains some five days and then found myself once again entering the village of Sidi

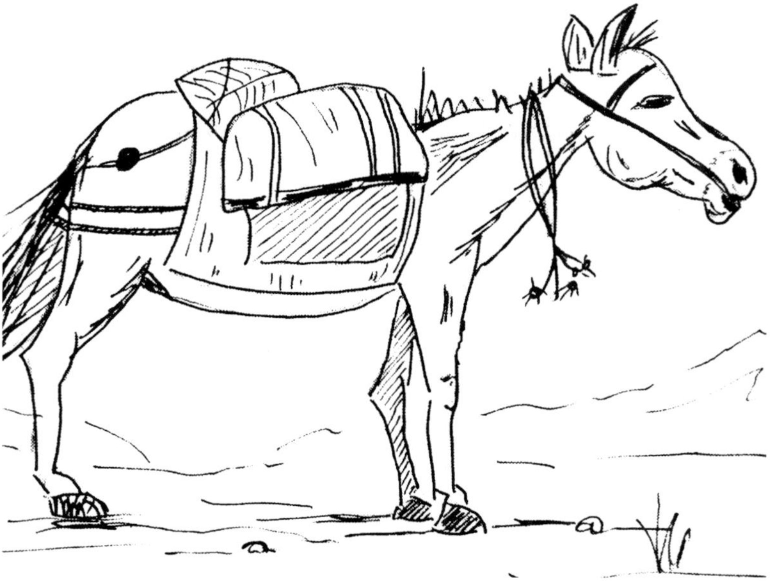

THE UNCOMPLAINING MULE

No story of the Atlas mountains would be complete without paying homage to the mules. These beasts of burden toil from dawn to dusk up and down the mountain passes taking mountaineers and their equipment up into the mountains. They form a valuable source of income to the muleteers. They are kept together in the village usually under the shade of the walnut groves. They are docile, uncomplaining and to the expeditions doctor may serve as an ambulance.

Chamharouch. The villagers came out to meet us and Ali was there beaming at us as we approached. He took me to his home and we sat on the floor and once again drank mint tea. His house was small, comprising only two rooms, and faced onto the path that leads through the village. The front of his house was a shop selling beads and necklaces and I bought one of each. Before I left I gave him my sheath knife and started my journey down to Imlil. 'Good-bye Bonne Chance' I said to him. 'I hope our paths meet once again.' They were to do so when I returned to the High Atlas in 1988 on yet another expedition.

On my second visit some thirteen years later I once again found myself entering the village of Sidi Chamharouch. We walked into the village and sat down on the path drinking Coca Cola as we had done all those years before. I eventually approached some of the villagers and asked them for the whereabouts of Ali ben Braheim and even mentioned his mule, Sirdun. There was considerable confusion and nobody seemed to really understand what I was talking about. I turned towards Peter, sat down and we bought another drink. About ten minutes later a small man appeared, I did not recognise him nor he me but I believed it was Ali ben Braheim. 'I am the doctor,' I said and pointed to his wrist and head and once again that magical smile appeared on his face and he flung his arms round me and started shaking me vigorously by the hand. There was no doubt this was Ali. Our paths had met once more and he took me to his home. We sat on the same floor and again we drank mint tea together. I understood on talking to him that he was married and had two children and that life had been reasonably kind to him. Peter took our photographs standing outside his home. I left him my cigarettes and lighter and he followed us out of the village as we once again continued our journey.

On my second visit to the mountains I did not climb Toubkal again. I made sure everything in the camp was in order and after two days had to return to Imlil, where I looked after the camp there.

THE NIGHT I FAILED TO TURN UP

It was about four o'clock on a Saturday afternoon when a message came down from the upper camp to state that one of the scouts had broken his ankle. Larsen, the headman of the village, was duly summoned and with my medical gear packed into the panniers of one of the mules and in the company of two Berber muleteers I again started on the long journey to the Neltner Hut. I told Larsen and Peter that I was determined to return later that night.

As far as I could understand Larsen was responsible for controlling everything that happened in Imlil. He was in his thirties and, like his father before him, had been a mountain guide. He unfortunately had a marked stammer and a facial twitch. He was, however, a man of considerable intelligence and spoke French and English that he had presumably learned when he was a mountain guide. He was the co-ordinator between ourselves and the villagers and apparently could organise anything. He arranged meals for us, deals with the muleteers and was even capable of getting cigarettes if you were desperate for them. He was a most amazing, gentle and helpful man who was of great service to us during our stay. He was another person I would not forget on my travels as an expedition doctor. He took Peter and I to his home where we spent a pleasant hour discussing our plans with him. He was most co operative and helped to make our visit a success. It seemed to me that if you were in trouble and shouted for Larsen, he would suddenly appear and sort things out for you!

By the time I reached the Neltner Hut it was dark. Travelling along the narrow paths with steep drops down to the river was frightening. I could hear the river cascading down the mountains and wondered how far it was to the bottom. I can remember thinking that if the mule stumbled I would have had it! At the camp site everyone was asleep so I put a torch on my head and made the sound of an ambulance siren and soon the camp woke up! '"The Accy Quack" is here' someone remarked in the darkness! I was taken to the unfortunate youngster and thought he had probably broken his ankle, but the injury was not too serious. The ankle joint was stable but he was very tender around his ankle ligaments. I put his boot back on and strapped it up and found somewhere to spend the night. It was at this time I remembered I had told Larsen I would return that night but there was no way I was going back down again in the darkness.

The following day we perched the boy on the back of a mule and set off back to Imlil. There was no Ali ben Braheim in Sidi Chamharouch, which saddened me, and we plodded our way down the valley. We descended lower and lower and the temperature began to rise. As we reached the Plain of Arond the young boy started crying with pain, became hysterical and eventually passed out. There was no way this lad was going any further. Tears were rolling down his face when he was revived and he was very frightened and would have nothing to do with any of us. I asked two other members to go to Imlil, summon Larsen and return with a stretcher. Some two hours later they returned. I sedated my patient and then we carried him back to the camp. Here he was looked after by some of the aspiring nurses and was shown considerable care and attention. Gradually he appeared to recover from his ordeal but this proved later not to be the case.

The next day I met Larsen on the main path that leads through the village. 'Thank you' I said 'for sending the stretcher yesterday when we were in trouble.' He looked at me and there was a silence. 'I waited for you all night' he said. He had apparently left his home at about midnight and had walked with Peter to the Plain of Arond and there the two of them had spent the night waiting for my return. I felt very guilty, as I had definitely told them that I would return in the night. The guilt must have shown on my face and I repeated to him that I was sorry and explained what had happened. He looked at me and put his hand on my shoulder and smiled. 'I am glad he is well again' he said. 'So am I' I replied, but it did not make me feel any better.

The poor lad was still in a hopeless state of panic and distress and our journey back to Marrakesh three days later was not without its problems.

We said farewell to Larsen and some of the villagers and set off in the direction Asni with the idea of stopping at the Hotel Toubkal. Here we had a beer and enjoyed a swim in the pool but it was as we were leaving the boy again started crying and became hysterical once more. I sedated him again and we eventually arrived back at the school for the blind in Marrakesh. I spoke to Peter about his management and decided he should have his ankle X-rayed and also suggested he should be flown home as he was becoming quite poorly and showed no signs of calming down, despite all our efforts. This we agreed to do. Three of us took him to the casualty department at the hospital in Marrakesh.

This was not the best place on earth to receive treatment. There was blood on the floor and vomit in a corner and whole place put the fear of God into me. The minor ops room was a mess with old needles lying around and catgut still on the needle obviously waiting to be used again on the next unsuspecting victim. We were approached by a nurse and she agreed that the boy's ankle should be X-rayed. We then had to go and buy the X-ray plates and with these in our hands we returned to the casualty department. It was at this time that a crazed drug addict burst into the department and started fighting with anyone he could lay his hands on. Some of the porters grabbed him and, as fast as he had entered, he left. I was waiting for the young lad with the ankle injury to start up another outburst but fortunately he did not. Like us all, he was just mesmerised by the whole incident.

To my amazement the X-rays revealed that he had a badly broken ankle and the doctors said they were going to operate on him. I have seen some sights in my medical career and there was no way I was going to allow them to operate on him there so we agreed just to take him away without asking any more questions. We were about to do this when a surgeon arrived and I rapidly introduced myself to him He had another look at the X-rays and remarked that they had been taken from the wrong ankle and his ankle was not too badly injured. I could have kissed his feet but decided not to bother! It was with much relief that we left the hospital and returned to camp.

It was on the way back to the camp that I mentioned to the young scout the possibility of flying him home. It was the first time I had seen him smile in days. From being sullen and depressed his face lit up with relief. When he arrived back at the base camp he eagerly told his friends of his imminent return home. I did not ask Peter how he had arranged it but the following day we drove with him to Agadir Airport and the boy was flown home by courtesy of the Air Ambulance. If as a doctor you have to use this facility I can highly recommend it to you. He was shown every kindness during this return trip and when he had left I must confess we breathed a sigh of relief. Basically, he should never have been chosen to go on such an expedition, but I must confess I was glad it was not me that had injured my ankle climbing in the High Atlas Mountains.

This exercise brought home to me the problems that can face an expedition doctor in comparison with a general practitioner at home. In England, when faced with such a problem, it is just a question of picking up the telephone and having word with a hospital casualty officer and arranging his transport by ambulance. I was faced with a dangerous journey at night sitting on the back of a mule, sedating and comforting a hysterical patient and I will never forget our experiences at the hospital in Marrakesh and finally driving a whole day to the airport to enable him to be flown home. Such is the life of an expedition doctor!

THE OLD LADY AND THE DYING BABY

I had been in Imlil at the base camp for about two days after climbing Mount Toubkal. We were generally lazing about doing nothing and someone was starting to prepare lunch when Larsen came up walking briskly into the camp area. I thought he had come to check on things and make sure everything was in order. There is an elderly man from one of the outlying villages who is concerned about his wife and asked if the doctor would come and see if he could help. It is remarkable how quickly news travels in the mountains. 'Certainly,' I volunteered, grabbing my medical rucksack and also one of the venture guides who was interested in nursing. 'Where is he and how far is his village?'

'Follow me' replied Larsen and we were introduced to an elderly Berber who must have been in his sixties.

We followed him up the cobbled street that led through the village, passed by the tree where the village barber earnt his living and turned right just before the walnut groves where the mules were kept. The path turned off to the right and twisted and turned through fields of maize but soon we began to climb quite steeply. Eventually, after about half an hour, we reached another path that led to the old man's village. We could see it perched precariously on the steep mountainside.

As we approached the village we saw children playing on the path and cattle and hens largely blocked our path. The path ended in a small square dominated by a temple but just before we arrived here we were shown a small wooden door on the right hand side of the track. We duly entered. We found ourselves in a barn with cattle standing in hay while others were lying down. At the far end of the barn was a wooden staircase going up to the floor above. As we climbed the stairs we had to avoid the odd chicken but as we looked up there was a row of smiling children's faces, obviously very interested in their guests. Once up the stairs, we were escorted into a small room with a stone floor, a mirror on the wall a small carpet in the middle and a selection of cushions in the far corner. We were then left alone in our new surroundings. We waited for what appeared to be a long time, but eventually an elderly lady was helped into the room by two younger men who I presumed were her sons. They escorted her across the room and laid her down on the cushions at the far end of the room. We were then invited to examine her. My nurse for the day was asked to lift the woman's dress and that revealed a large infected, painful ulcer which I assumed was the result of an injury.

I opened my medical rucksack and instructed my nurse on how to clean and dress the ulcer. This she accomplished with great skill. I was impressed and told her so. Having finished the dressing and smiling at our patient I then gave her an injection of penicillin to aid her recovery. She smiled kindly at us both and thanked us and then with the assistance of her two sons left the room. Soon we were alone again, not knowing quite what to do. 'I bet this is a little different from college at home,' I remarked. 'I don't really know why I went to college to study teaching' she replied. 'I'm really interested in becoming a nurse.'

After about five minutes by which time we had tidied up, one of her sons entered the room carrying a tray of mint tea and we sat on the floor again to quench our thirst. We explained to him we would return in a couple of days to revisit his mum and look again at her wound. We thanked him for the tea and left the room. The kids were still there outside beaming at us, we dodged the occasional chicken on the stairs, swerved around the cows and found ourselves in the sunlit street outside. We sauntered along the path that had led us to the village and once again started to descend to the base camp far below. We arrived just in time to miss lunch!

Two days later we found ourselves in the same room after having managed to avoid the local hazards. Soon the elderly lady limped into the room on her own with her sons following behind. It seemed she was starting to get better. My nurse lifted her dress once again and skilfully removed the dressings to reveal that the ulcer was much better and obviously not causing as much pain. She redressed it, bandaged her up and I left some antibiotic powder along with more dressings and instructions as to how to look after the ulcer. We felt well pleased with our endeavours.

We were preparing to leave when a young mother with a child in her arms entered the room. The child was submerged under several blankets. Once we had removed these a small dehydrated dying child was revealed. I eagerly enquired from the son of the elderly lady what had happened to the child. It turned out that the baby was suffering from gastroenteritis. I explained the seriousness of the situation to him and explained we would take both the mother and the baby to Marrakesh where we were heading later that day. This the young mother refused to do despite our protestations and offer of help. The child needed urgent hospital admission and drip therapy if it was going to make it and even then it would be touch and go. Once again we tried to persuade her to come with us but to no avail. I stripped the child and examined it. Apart from severe dehydration the child also had pneumonia. I gave her some electrolyte and antibiotic powder as a gesture and then she collected her baby and left the room after thanking us. Before we finally left we drank more tea and soon found ourselves outside on the path of the village. The mood was very different to our last visit. The young would-be nurse was in tears. 'I am definitely going to become a nurse' she wept, 'and what is more I'm coming back here. I cannot believe what I have seen.' I put my arm around her to try and comfort her. 'There is one thing we can do' I suggested 'and that is to contact Larsen to see if he can persuade them to go to hospital.' 'Don't bother' she exploded 'it will probably die anyway.' The whole occasion was one of helplessness and distress. We walked the remaining journey down to the base camp in silence and then I went off to find Larsen.

Later, when we were packing up to leave in the direction of Marrakesh, Peter tapped me on my arm and pointed to a line of patients sitting on a wall in the main street. 'That looks like your afternoon surgery' he laughed. Two of the children had coughs and colds; one young girl had burned her arm which needed dressing and the little fellow at the end wanted some cigarettes. Instead, we gave him some sweets and he ran off, obviously happy with his prize. We soon finished packing, loaded our belongings onto the vans, said farewell to Larsen and headed off in the direction of Asni which led us to the road to Marrakesh.

The incident of the elderly lady and the baby left with a feeling of distress and impotence. Certainly one of our patients was getting better but the same could not be said for the other. This was the first time I was faced with leaving a dying child in its mother's arms but it was obvious to me that there was nothing else I could do. I certainly could not kidnap the child and run off with it to hospital, I had to leave it where it was. I do not know what the infant mortality is in these remote mountain Berber villages, but it must be high. I tried to console myself by remembering the happy smiling faces of the young children standing on the veranda. At least they had made it and were obviously fit and healthy. I suppose up to a point it did.

KENYA

NAIROBI

Kenya is a country of many contrasts, not only in the environment but also in relation to the wide numbers of people who live there. There are deserts and mountains with Alpine snows, forests, woodlands and open plains. There are vast freshwater lakes and superb beaches on the coast. It is bounded to the north by the high mountains of Ethiopia and in the northeast by the semi-desert of Somaliland. On the eastern border is a glorious coastline with beaches and modern day hotels which attract many thousands of tourists every year. To the south lies Tanzania and to the west is Uganda. In the north the land is low-lying and semi-desert and this forms the largest part of Kenya. It supports relatively few people who exist with their camels, goats and sheep. It is to this part of Kenya that we were heading to embark on a camel trek with the Gabbra tribe in the Huri Hills on the Kenyan-Ethiopian border. To the east lies a different land, well watered from the monsoon rains that sweep in from the Indian Ocean. The land there is lush and fertile and supports a wide range of agriculture and farming. To the south and west are higher grounds which are split from north to south by the great Rift Valley system. This starts far north in Israel and ends even further south in Botswana. On the eastern part of the Rift Valley lies Mount Kenya and rainfall is plentiful at certain times of the year. The land there is also productive and forms one of the bread baskets of the country. On the west side of the Rift Valley are the peaks of the Mau ranges and here again the land is fertile but most of the water there comes not from the Indian Ocean but from Lake Victoria.

The first people in inhabit Kenya were the bushmen and as before they were pushed out from their original lands by further tribes. Tribes first spread in from today, what is Ethiopia and Somaliland probably about some five thousand years ago. Three thousand years ago they were joined by the Bantu from the south and others from the north, probably from the region of the Nile. The most recent arrivals in Kenya were the Galla that the Gabbra are descended from.

While all this activity was going on inland, the coast was not without its changes. All along the east coast of Africa traders from the Far East arrived, mainly the Arabs and Persians. This is the reason why the largely Islamic culture developed and still persists today. It is the mixture of Arab and African blood that gave rise to the Swahili tribe.

Great changes occurred in Kenya when man decided to adorn himself and his home with ivory and the demand for ivory soared. As this happened so trading caravans set forth from the coast inland and the horrendous trade in ivory began. The consequences of this are still being felt today and in the eyes of many the battle against the ivory poacher is being lost.

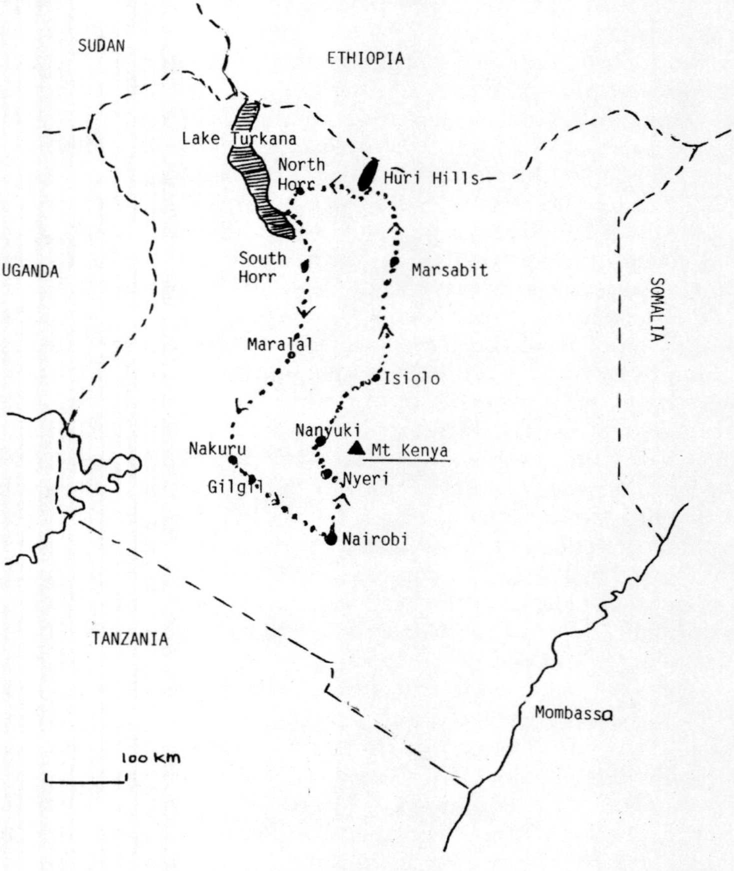

JOURNEY THROUGH KENYA

In 1850 Kenya was run by the British and they developed a rapid communications system which was organised to run trade and commerce more efficiently. In 1896 the British decided to build a railway from the coast at Mombasa to the interior, hoping to reach Lake Victoria. This was the birth of the Mombasa-Nairobi Railway. This led to the emergence of Nairobi as a city and there was a steady influx of Europeans into Kenya and the now modern agricultural economy started and progressed. However, there were many problems with the local tribes especially the Kikuyu, and this eventually erupted into The Mau Mau revolt and later the independence of Kenya.

In 1963 Kenya became independent of British rule but a large white community remained and the economic growth of Kenya continued to progress, especially in agriculture. Today Kenya is a major exporter of tea, coffee and fruit. The economy has also been boosted by the tourist trade and this has exceeded all their expectations. But there are conservationists who now believe this should be restricted because the ecology is suffering as a result of too many people entering a sensitive environment.

Kenya is probably one of the most stable communities in Africa at the moment but it still has a one-party state. As I write this book there is unrest amongst the student population and they are demanding a more democratic structure in Kenya. The first president of Kenya was Jomo Kenyatta, an outstanding politician, and his policies are still being carried out today under the presidency of Daniel Arap Moi. The way things are progressing from a political point of view it will probably not be long before democratic elections take place as they have done in Zambia.

I visited Kenya in 1990 and travelled both north and south. We visited the Amboseli and Masai Mara game parks, spent some time in Nairobi, but most of our trip was spent in the far north in the former Northern Frontier district of Kenya. After heading north to the Huri Hills we embarked on a camel trek for two weeks, crossed the Chalbi desert, visited Lake Turkana and then returned to Nairobi. The whole expedition lasted some five weeks. We saw the wide range of countryside scenery that exists, came into contact with several of the tribes and the whole experience was one that I will never forget. I can well understand why so many people feel the need to return to this most beautiful country.

Nairobi came into existence when the British built the Mombasa-Nairobi railway. The original idea was to reach Lake Victoria a distance of some 570 miles. At first there was little in the way of trouble as the gradient was favourable but as this became more difficult there were more and more problems. When they reached what is now Nairobi they decided to call a temporary halt. The land was suitable for building, marshalling yards and there was ample land to build houses and accommodation for the workers. It was not long before they decided to move the main depot from Mombasa to Nairobi to deal with the problems at first hand. As Nairobi developed, commercial enterprise followed and the original shanty town grew at a rapid rate. The so-called Lunatic Line cost the British Government several million pounds, an enormous sum of money in those days, and to recoup some of the money the line was used to carry freight. The government encouraged white settlers to come to Kenya with the promise of cheap land, but although the idea was good, the organisation was poor and there was a higher than expected influx of settlers. This caused many problems with the local tribes, especially the Kikuyu, and resulted in inter-racial resentment which persisted for many years and was never really resolved. Apart from the Europeans there was also the problem of the arrival of many Indians at the same time. The two groups competed with one another for trade and development and neither paid any attention to the views or needs of the local Africans. As time progressed, however, there was a switch of power in favour of the indigenous Africans.

Nairobi became a cosmopolitan city and this is manifested by the different numbers of religions that are present. There are mosques, temples, churches and synagogues and also different cultural and tribal races apart from the Europeans, including Arabs, Indians, Pakistanis, Japanese and Somalis. The most numerous Africans found in Nairobi are the Kikuyu, but this is not surprising as Nairobi stands on the borders of their tribal lands. With all this diverse population and activity, Nairobi developed and expanded rapidly as a commercial centre. The population also escalated; over a million people live here and the rocketing population is of great concern to the government. Many people in Nairobi find themselves without homes or jobs.

The base camp for the expedition in Nairobi was at Hillcrest School, which is just up the road from the main gates of the Nairobi Game Park in the southern part of Nairobi. It is a modern school run on the British system of education and teaches a wide range of students of differing nationalities. The buildings and classrooms are of a high standard and sporting activities are obviously encouraged. There is a swimming pool, tennis courts as well as cricket and rugby pitches. Many of the pupils take the equivalent of A level and then enter university life in England. We stayed here for three days before we started our journey north. We used the facilities of the kitchens, slept in various classrooms and obviously used the swimming pool. However, the water was not as warm as it was tempting! The journey to the city centre took about twenty minutes.

Entering Nairobi by car was an education in itself; three lines of traffic moving slowly towards the city centre in the morning rush hour. So snail-like was the traffic that local Africans were able to sell newspapers, magazines and even pictures to the slow-moving traffic. The skyline is dominated by huge office blocks built of glass and concrete, dominated by the Kenyatta Conference Centre. It is a modern busy city with modern facilities, including first-class hotels and many shops. The Arabs tend to own the shops whilst the Africans run the markets.

Eating in Nairobi is superb and on my arrival I was taken by Peter to the Norfolk Hotel for lunch. There we ate steak and kidney and cottage pie as well as sampling other local dishes on our subsequent visits. In the middle of the hotel is an enchanting courtyard with well kept gardens onto which face some of the hotel bedrooms. The hotel also has its own tourist shop. We also visited the Muthiaga Club which featured in the film Out of Africa. It was here that the early explorers planned their expeditions before setting off into the bush. The meeting place for those shopping or sightseeing was usually the New Stanley Hotel on a table near the famous thorn tree. It was on this tree that messages have been left for decades and still are today. The food here was also good, especially the Indian style, with a variety of curries and spices. After the expedition had once again returned to Nairobi, towards the day or our return home, we spent an enjoyable evening at the Carnivore restaurant, where we gorged ourselves on steak, giraffe and zebra. After we had eaten our fill we spent the rest of the evening in the disco.

Apart from trying to eat our way through Nairobi we also visited other places of interest! I spent the afternoon at the National Museum and snake park. The former is well worth a visit, although fairly expensive to enter if you are a visitor, but well worth the money as there is much to see. Many tribal and zoological exhibits are on show, along with many fine exhibits of art work. There is also a well documented paleontology department giving an account of the emergence of man. Much of this work has been carried out near the shores of Lake Turkana by Richard Leakey whom Peter met in his office at the Nairobi Game Park. I spent a very enjoyable couple of hours wandering around looking at the exhibits. In the adjoining grounds to the museum is the Snake Park but I found this disappointing. Sure there were many snakes to see along with amusing notices telling you not to feed the snakes, but it had obviously been visited by many people and it showed. The whole place could have done with a good clean. We paid a visit to the Game Park just down the road from the school and it was strange to see giraffe and wild game against the backdrop of the Nairobi skyline.

I was fortunate to visit the civilian airport in Nairobi and had an unforgettable trip down the Rift Valley to Lake Magadi on the Tanzanian border. We flew down the valley and over the lake with its flocks of flamingos and landed on a small runway in the bush. During the flight I was asked if I would like to take the controls and so I could not resist flying low over the lake to watch the flamingos take off. The landing in the bush was complicated by baboons on the runway but we managed to miss them! We walked to the edge of the Rift Valley and I felt quite humble to be in such magnificent surroundings. My host for the day was Joe O'Brien, the Irish Consul General in Nairobi, with his Piper Cherokee aircraft. On the way back I asked if we could fly low over a hill on the outskirts of Nairobi which had a steep drop on the other side. I lined the aircraft up and we skimmed over the hill. The excitement was too much for me and my hands left the controls and I let out a shriek of delight. To my surprise, the aircraft did not deviate one inch and I realised he had been flying the plane all the time! We both split our sides laughing, but I never really forgave him! Having landed, I was taken to the bar and there we sat drinking beer and chewing billtong. It was at the airport that the Flying Doctor Service was initiated and on our trip we paid to use the facilities should we have required them. Fortunately, we didn't but it was a close-run thing and that story I will relate later.

Driving in Nairobi is not without its problems. In the city centre the speed you can obtain is obviously limited but we did witness one accident as we sat drinking beer one evening at the bar in the New Stanley Hotel. Fortunately, nobody was seriously injured but there was quite a commotion. One of the passengers had a badly cut face and a fight nearly broke out between the drivers, each blaming the other. Driving in the suburbs, especially at night is a different story from daytime and not without its risks. The roads tend to be in a poor state of repair and drivers at night seem to have little regard for other road users. There was also the problem of police checkpoints. Heavy steel spiked bars prevented any further passage along the road and the police were armed with automatic weapons. We had little trouble with them, but once again common sense and doing exactly as you were told were essential.

We visited several European homes during our stay and all were heavily secured with elaborate alarm systems. High fences and locked gates were the order of the day. Large dogs roamed free in the gardens and barked loudly at any noise or disturbance. Some of the houses had steel doors and bars at the windows. I heard from Peter that some of the older residents still slept with a loaded pistol under their pillows.

Whilst in Nairobi I was fortunate, to talk to the wife of a local European who was doing research into Sleeping Sickness. At one time this disease had decimated Africa and in the early part of this century, over a million deaths occurred in the Congo alone. In one outbreak around Lake Victoria 200,000 people out of a population of 300,000 died within eight years. It is still a major problem. Today much of the research control has been the victim of other national priorities which have involved military expenditure but also corruption and complacency. These have eroded the public health foundations in many African nations and as a result Sleeping Sickness has resurfaced as a major threat. Briefly, it is transmitted by the bite of the Tsetse fly and the trypanosome, a protozoan, enters the body. There is an indurated area at the site of the bite followed by a high fever and facial swelling. The parasite then attacks mainly the central nervous system with devastating effects and sometimes death. Specific treatment is, however, completely successful. The East African disease primarily affects those who live in or enter the game-inhabited woodland or bush. The presence of an infection can rapidly depopulate a river valley and the risks of disease prevent vast fertile areas from being cultivated. Such waste of land is disastrous in tropical areas where malnutrition causes so much infant mortality and debility in adults. It is largely controlled by removing the environment in the bush where the tsetse fly lives. She was fascinating to talk to and I enjoyed listening to the problems with which she is faced, which are so different to public health matters in this country.

I then discussed with her the object of our expedition and remarked that we were going to visit Lake Turkana in the north. Her face lit up and she then told me the risks of Hydatid disease, which is another parasitic disease involving a tape-worm that uses both dogs and man as hosts. She told me that the highest incidence of this condition was in the Lake Turkana district and that the human infection rate reaches between five and ten per cent. It was at this time that I was beginning to wish I had stopped at home! The cysts of the tape-worm are passed in the stools of the dog and pass to humans in a variety of ways. First of all, to children crawling on the floor who accidentally put their hands in the dog excreta and then transfer it to their mouths, but also in adults from the women who wear heavy jewellery around their necks and to stop it rubbing against their necks, they protect themselves by rubbing a mixture of camel fat and dog excreta on their bodies. The Turkana do not bury their dead and their bodies are left to rot and decay. They are sometimes eaten by dogs and this is one of the ways the tape-worm passes back to the dog. Having learned this information I gave another talk with members of the expedition about the risks involved.

On our journey through Kenya we saw many contrasting ways of life; from the relative comfort of Nairobi to the poor, remote and simple ways of life predominant in the tribal communities in the north. Here life proceeds as it has done for centuries and there has been little in the way of progress. I contemplated the happiness of these two extremes. It was obvious to me that the more content were the people who had little in the way of wealth or possessions. Their simple life and needs seemed to be satisfied, although they had obvious hardships but greed and the excessive attainment of wealth did not erode their charm and generosity. Crime is low in tribal communities and they all pull together for the common good; the same is obviously not true in Nairobi.

I hope to return to Kenya in three years time as a doctor on another expedition, this time around the shores of Lake Turkana - I cannot wait. I suppose to some people golf and other activities are addictive but to me expedition medicine certainly is.

THE HURI HILLS

I once again found myself following in the footsteps of Peter Drake on another expedition, the purpose of which was to travel to northern Kenya, meet up with the Gabbra tribe and then embark on a camel trek for fourteen days in the Huri Hills and Chalbi Desert. We set off from Nairobi having stayed for a few days at Hillcrest School where we had organised our final plans. All the gear and water supply were sorted out and early one morning we departed in two trucks driven by local Africans. The trucks were in a doubtful state of repair but we were assured they would complete their task and return us later to Nairobi.

We headed north towards Nyeri and then passed Mount Kenya. Here we stayed for a short time in one of the game lodges and had a beer and a rest. The next stop was a Nanyuki where the Equator crosses Africa - it was a popular place to take photographs. We visited the grave of Baden Powell on our journey that day and by evening camped just south of Isiolo in the bush. This was my first night in the African bush and one I will never forget. The scenery was stunning, with the peaks of Mount Kenya in the distance. Soon after leaving Isiolo we reached Archers Crossing on the Southern border of the Chalbi Desert where we were halted by a police check-point. To go any further we had to go in convoy or take an armed guard with us. Seated in the back of each truck was a young, armed soldier who accompanied us to Marsabit. They were obviously concerned about our safety. After a long journey through the desert we entered Marsabit in the late afternoon where darkness was rapidly setting in. We camped the night in the Marsabit National Park. That night I found frightening and disturbing and the whole expedition was in a state of unrest. The area we camped in was a small clearing in the bush surrounded by high trees. The noises in the night were unnerving and I was glad to see daylight once again. I was not sorry to see the back of the Marsabit and we once again proceeded north across the Chalbi Desert hoping to reach a small Gabbra settlement at Karabara by evening. During the day the mood of the expedition improved again and the progress we made was good. Towards late afternoon we approached Karabara and then disaster struck. One of the local African drivers had been nicknamed Ayrton Senna by some of the members, and it was he who smashed the back axle of his truck as we drew close to the village. We decided that two of us should try to reach Karabara, as we had been led to believe that there may have been transport there. Fortunately, a passing Landrover was heading in that direction and two of us asked for a lift. Soon after leaving we were confronted by another vehicle heading towards the site of our accident, the driver of which was Andersen, the man we had come to meet and who was the go-between for us in our dealings with the Gabbra. We changed vehicles and set off back. The poor driver was in a terrible state of panic and regret but had successfully halted our progress by his reckless driving.

Andersen was an American missionary working with the Gabbra. A huge man with a commanding voice, who obviously was in control of events in the village. He lived there with his family and we met his daughter who was travelling with him that day. She was in her late teens and on holiday from university life in America. We all stood around the abandoned truck and after he had inspected it Andersen said that it would have to stay there the night but the next day he thought he could repair it! I nearly fell off my perch. Here we were, miles away from anywhere, and he had the facilities to repair it! I was flabbergasted. 'You cannot stay here' he said, apparently because there were lions around and one of the villagers had been attacked and killed some months before. Needless to say, we rapidly collected our gear off the truck and eventually reached the mission house in Karabara where we spent the night. 'I hope you see a lion roar' he remarked 'there is a dust storm six feet in front of its mouth.' I distinctly remember thinking that I hoped we did not!

The mission house we stayed in at Karabara was substantially built with several rooms; there was a water supply from an underground well. The toilet facilities were at the end of a path in the garden and the views from the garden looked out to the Huri Hills - it was a most restful and peaceful place. This was the place Andersen had arranged for us to meet the Gabbra tribesmen who were to accompany us on our journey.

The next day late in the morning they duly arrived with their camels. There were two for each member; one for carrying the personal gear and the other for carrying water. The object was to travel in a circle through the hills, refill our water supply at an armed water dump that Andersen had organised and return to the mission house. The day after that we would walk across the Chalbi Desert and then to another Gabbra village at Kalacha and there the camel trek would end. With the help of the tribesmen we loaded the camels and were ready to set off about mid-afternoon. We walked for about three hours and then set up our camp. On our way we came across a wild camel and one idiot shouted 'walkies!' and the camel started to follow us! Needless to say, the walk continued at a brisk pace until the poor camel had had enough and wandered off again. We walked for twelve days covering over a hundred and ten miles before we finally reach Kalacha.

Each day would start at sunrise, after a drink and helping to load the gear on the camels, we set off walking. We walked through the bush until about lunch time, stopping roughly every hour for a drink and to admire the spectacular scenery. Peter would find an acacia tree and there we would wait until the camels caught us up and make camp for the night. All the water was collected and accounted for and after a short rest and something to eat we spent the afternoon relaxing. Ornithologists list-

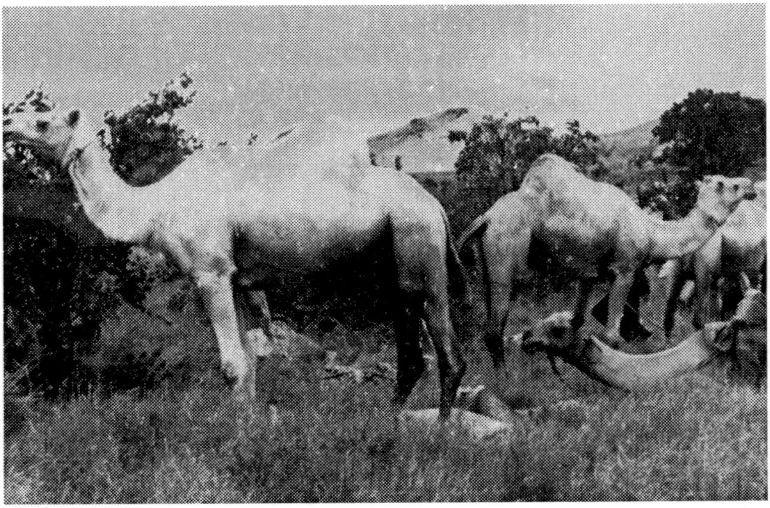

CAMELS IN THE HURI HILLS

ed birds they had seen and even tried to catch them in nets; artists sketched; zoologists set traps for small mammals and sound recordists also were kept busy. It was absolutely magical to be in such a remote and wild place.

The idea that when walking through the African bush wild animals are around every corner and snakes hang from the trees is simply not true. We saw relatively little game but the bird life was spectacular. One day the Gabbra became very excited when they found both leopard and lion tracks around the camp but fortunately we did not encounter them. At night jackals would come near to the camp but they did not pose any problem. We saw two cobras which we avoided, but there was plenty of evidence of snakes around in the form of discarded skins. I spent many a happy hour collecting porcupine quills, but, again, did not see any. We occasionally met Gabbra shepherds with their sheep and goats and one night they camped with the camel herders. At night they collected bushes and made a small corral for their goats. We tried to buy one of the goats to eat one evening but they were not willing to sell us one.

As evening approached the evening meal was prepared around the fire. We had taken dehydrated food with us. After the meal was finished and the camp tidied up we would sit around the fire talking and chatting into the night. It was at this time the Gabbra would come into our camp and I was kept busy looking after their pains and complaints. I really could not find much the matter with them most of the time, but still gave them tablets which would do them any harm, though on the other hand would not do them much good either. I soon changed my method of treatment and gave them injections instead so from then on trade rapidly declined! One of the girls had been on previous expeditions where each member at times like this was given five minutes to tell the others all about themselves in their allotted time. This proved to be a most instructive and sometimes alarming exercise. We had trouble stopping one young scout from talking, as what he was going to do to his brother when he returned was nobody's business! It is amazing to be in such a remote place where people's minds become so open and problems that have troubled them for years become so apparent to them. It was a most enlightening facet of human behaviour.

After the talking people wandered back to their sleeping bags and the watch during the night began. The fire was kept burning all night and the watch changed every hour. Before the Gabbra went to sleep they would sing and chant around their fire. One night they allowed us to tape one of their songs as we sat in the black night, huddled around their fire. The skies were clear at night and the stars were bright and distinct. One member spent most of his evenings trying to identify them and teach us something about the celestial heavens. I am afraid much of his seed fell on stony ground as far as I was concerned!

The Huri Hills are in the northern territory of Kenya and are small and dome-shaped. It is a wild and desolate area and, although you do not see much in the way of game, you are aware that eyes are watching you. It is certainly not a place for fools. It was here many years ago that the early explorers came, but from the north, not as we had done from the south. Delamere was one of the better known and he used Mount Feroli as a reference point as we were doing. When walking through the bush the whole party had to be kept together with nobody lagging behind at the back. If this happened our guide would stop until they had caught up. Nothing disastrous happened on our trek but the night we spent at the water dump was unsettling and not without its problems. It was here that the Gabbra decided they were not going any further the next day as we were told their camels were tired. After lengthy diplomacy the problem was resolved. The camp had a strange atmosphere about it; there were snakes around and jackals were numerous around the fire at night. The whole experience had been unpleasant.

The days seemed endless in the bush and I have seldom felt

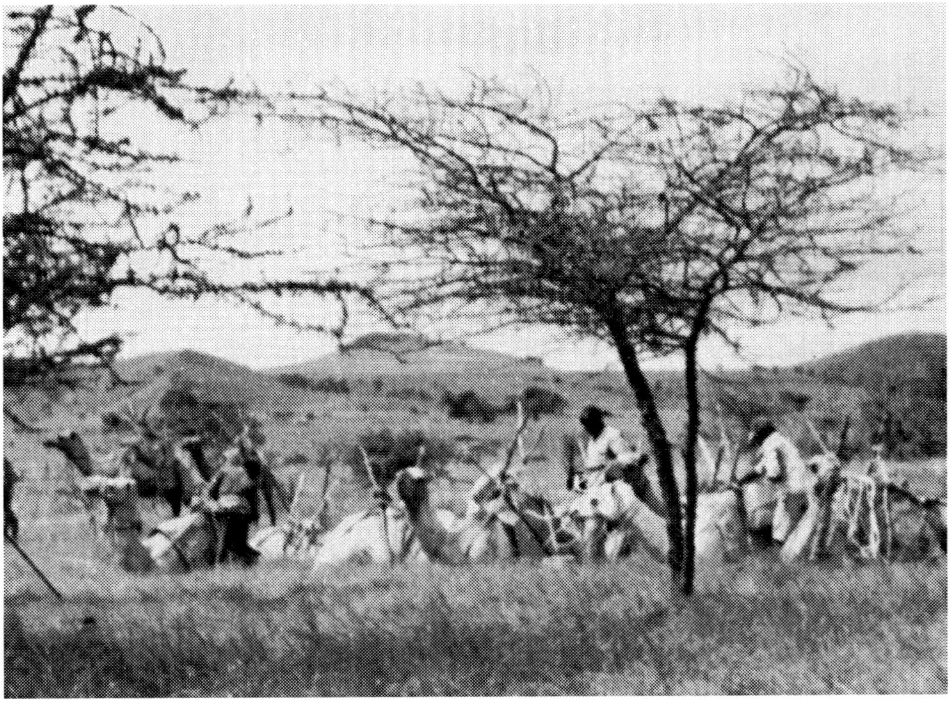

CAMELS BEING UNLOADED AT THE END OF THE DAYS MARCH
(The containers carried our water supply)

so relaxed and at peace with myself. It is a wonderful place to contemplate your life and problems and enables you to obtain a more clear insight into them. All the problems you have seem to become easier to deal with . The main problem we had was with water, as if this ran out we would be in serious trouble. It was not the gas or electric bill that posed the problems, it was more a question of survival. It was an ideal place to put things into their correct perspective. Water was at a premium and we did not wash for twelve days, though even that did not seem to matter. Once you were dirty that was that and to hell with it!

The Gabbra camel herders wore a mixture of local clothes and some had a more European form of dress. To watch them loading the camels in the morning was instructive. Two sticks at the front and two at the back all skilfully tied together with rope to form a framework. To this our gear and water were tied. Each of them carried his own spear and they followed us each day to

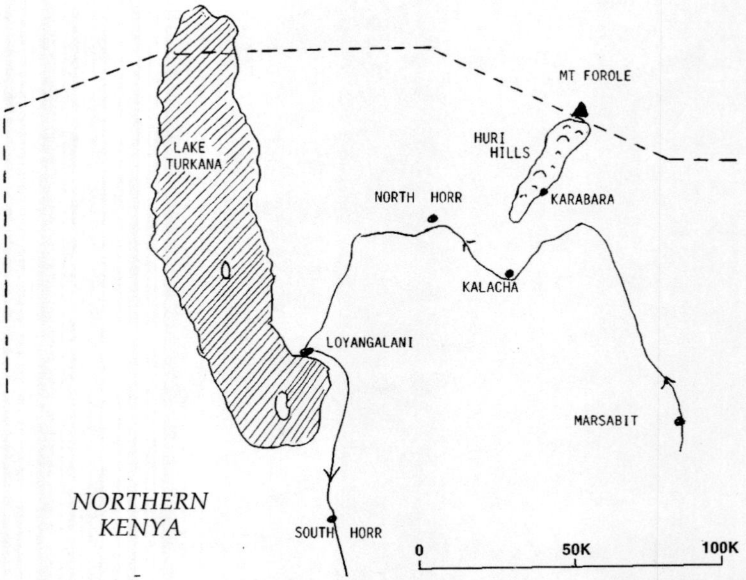

where we had decided to camp. On their arrival we would help them to unload and then they would let their camels graze in the bush and collect them together in the evening. They made camp at night about a hundred yards away from us, would light their fire and eat their meal, which we often supplemented. They used the goat skins and sticks to make a shelter at night. One goat skin formed the floor; they put their sticks in a line by the skin and another goat skin was used to form protection against the wind. The performance was finished off by sticking their spears into the ground. Later at night they huddled up in a blanket and went to sleep. How simple and how effective, I remember thinking. However, these people were not easy to relate to and tended to keep themselves to themselves. Any communication was primitive but they were very able to let us know when they wanted something. As I have found out before in remote areas, once people realise there is a doctor available they are very keen to seek medical advice. They had a leader who was referred to as the trade union man and it was he who was the spokesman for them. Not altogether a pleasant individual with a surly smile and certainly not a person to be trusted. Having said that we had no trouble with them on the journey but at the end of the camel trek there was a problem regarding their payment. This had been agreed in advance but an argument broke out regarding where they money was to be paid and even then they tried to obtain more. The main culprit was the trade union leader but eventually, and not without some trouble, the situation was resolved.

After ten glorious days of wandering through the bush we eventually returned to the mission house at Karabara late one afternoon. Here we had the luxury of a wash and a change of clothes. We retired to bed early that night as we had an early start the next day when our objective was to reach Kalacha. This turned out to be a day I will never forget.

We were up at first light, had a drink, loaded our gear onto the camels and set off following our Gabbra guide. As the morning progressed the temperature rose rapidly and by lunch time it was obvious that we had become lost. We had been assured that the journey to Kalacha could easily be done in a day and so we decided to carry on. As the temperature rose the pace began to fall off and members of the group started to feel the effects of travelling in the intense heat. The main problem was the psychological aspect; although people were tired and weary they also became despondent and the mood of the treck became low. At one stop I organised a golf match in the desert. We found a stick and collected some stones and whoever hit the stone the furthest won. They did not actually win anything but at least had the satisfaction of winning the first golf competition in the Chalbi desert. We collected ourselves together again and set off on our weary journey. By late afternoon, after walking since sunrise, we came across some acacia trees and the Gabbra guide became quite excited and realised where he was, the excitement in him was reflected in relief on our part! The Gabbra guide had been nicknamed Bruce by the members, but at the end of that day it had changed, though unfortunately what it was I cannot relate to you! We then had the problem of the following camels, as presumably they had become lost as well, but about an hour later we spotted them in the distance. The mood in the party changed again and people started laughing once more and conversation increased rapidly. That night we sat by the fire after our meal and reflected on the events of the day. The general opinion was that we were just glad to be safe and sound once again. The day had been arduous in the extreme but was finished off with a spectacular sunset. Our guide who had fallen from grace assured us that Kalacha was only a few hours away. I do not think many of us believed him!

The next day we once again set off and soon came across the track that eventually led us to Kalacha. It was late morning when we arrived and I felt like a million dollars. The depression of the day before rebounded and we marched at a brisk pace into the village. As we drew closer we came across small Gabbra settlements, and it was a relief to see signs of life again! As we entered the village we found ourselves on a runway and on the right-hand side of this stood a large acacia tree where we pitched camp. It was like heaven and the mood of the expedition rose even higher when we found there was a supply of cool beer! Later that afternoon when the camp had been sorted out Peter decided to hold a service under the acacia tree. One of the Kenyan scouts recited the "Lord's Prayer" in Swahili, there was a reading from the Bible and then we sang "The Day Thou Gavest Lord Is Ended." It nearly had the day before! It was a most moving ceremony and one I will never forget. I have never been an active Christian in my attendance at church but I certainly felt close the Creator that day.

IT'S HARD WORK BEING A DAD

I have been involved for many years now in expedition medicine and have travelled to remote and exciting places. I regard myself as being very fortunate but I have always been reluctant to leave home, especially as the day of departure looms closer. I worry about leaving my family and then worry about them when I am away. As the time comes to return home I cannot wait to see my kids again. I just love them.

My younger daughter Claire dropped several hints that one day she would like to join me on a trip and eventually her chance came. She travelled with me to northern Kenya in the Huri Hills. I had warned her that she would be treated like any other member of the trip and would have to make her own way. She would shown no favours from me and would have to stand on her own two feet.

During our trek in the Huri Hills the idea was that there would be two groups travelling in different directions but would meet up later after about ten days. One group would go in an anti-clockwise direction and the other clockwise and there would obviously be a time when they would cross after about five days. My daughter was travelling in the other group and not with me.

As the day approached when we would cross I could not help but be concerned as to how she would be. Our path took us to remote and potentially hostile places.

On the fifth day we saw the other party approaching - the

leaders at the front with the Gabbra guide - the rest following and the camels bringing up the rear carrying the water and equipment. As we grew closer I realised all was not well with my daughter. I knew this emotion well and had experienced it before when I realised my kids were in trouble. The doctor in charge of her group told me of his concern for her - she was not eating and undoubtedly struggling with her task. The implications were obvious. I stood in front of her and I am still not sure who was speaking but it had obviously been me. That must sound strange - it was. 'You have to carry on,' I explained to her - 'you must carry on; it's no use making me an excuse since if I were not here you would have no alternative.'

She turned away from my gaze but the look on her face confirmed my fears and she walked slowly back to her party to continue her part of the trek. I have never felt so wretched in my life. I did not console her and in retrospect she must have found that harsh indeed but the rules had been made before we left home and I was not about to change them. The emotions of parents are often put to severe testing indeed and this was one of those occasions.

I watched them slowly disappear from view into the bush and my mind was in torment for the next few days. That night I had great trouble sleeping and had an incredible urge to go to try to find her and tell her how much I loved her. I knew it was totally unrealistic so consoled myself through knowing well the people who were in charge of her group and the help of a night time drink of brandy. If I could not look after her I knew they would.

It was six days later we finally met up again as we entered the village of Kalacha. My daughter had arrived the day before with her group and had set up camp under an acacia tree beside the runway. I purposely waited at the back of our group as we entered the village to see if I could see her and have some time to assess how she was. I stood there trying to contain my emotions. She saw me and came rushing up to present me with a bottle of beer kept cool in a wet sock. My daughter knows me well! 'Sorry,' she explained, 'I had felt awful but soon recovered and enjoyed the rest of the trip.' As I looked down at her smiling face I could have hit her, reflecting on the emotions I had endured but decided not to bother and gave her a love. 'Come on' she said 'I will do your washing!'

Being a parent is an onerous responsibility indeed. When your kids are young you can guide and direct them, but as they grow older they have to make their own way in life. There is a transitional period between childhood and becoming an adult and it is not always an easy passage for either child or dad. The strongest emotion is to try and protect them from hurt but one day they have to do it for themselves. I realise it is a part of growing up and maturing. I think that day as we both stood in the wild African bush miles away from civilisation that my daughter took the first steps into adulthood. All kids have to do it some day but for a parent it is difficult to allow them to do it on their own and not stick your oar in. That was the day when my daughter took the first steps to becoming an independent woman in her own right and I think she made it. I'm not sure whether I fully recovered from it though, and remember it vividly to this day!

THE GABBRA TRIBE

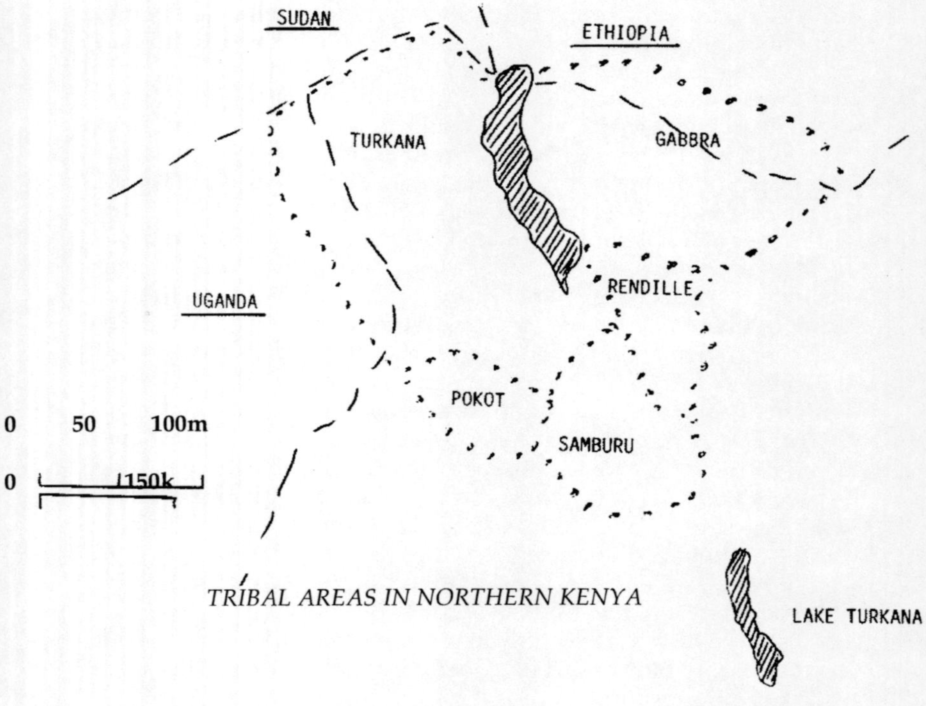

TRIBAL AREAS IN NORTHERN KENYA

Kalacha is a stable Gabbra community and like every other stable community in the desert depends on a supply of water. There was a bore hole at the far end of the village where they grew sugar cane and vegetables and camels used it as a watering hole. Peter is a genius at organisation as I have mentioned and

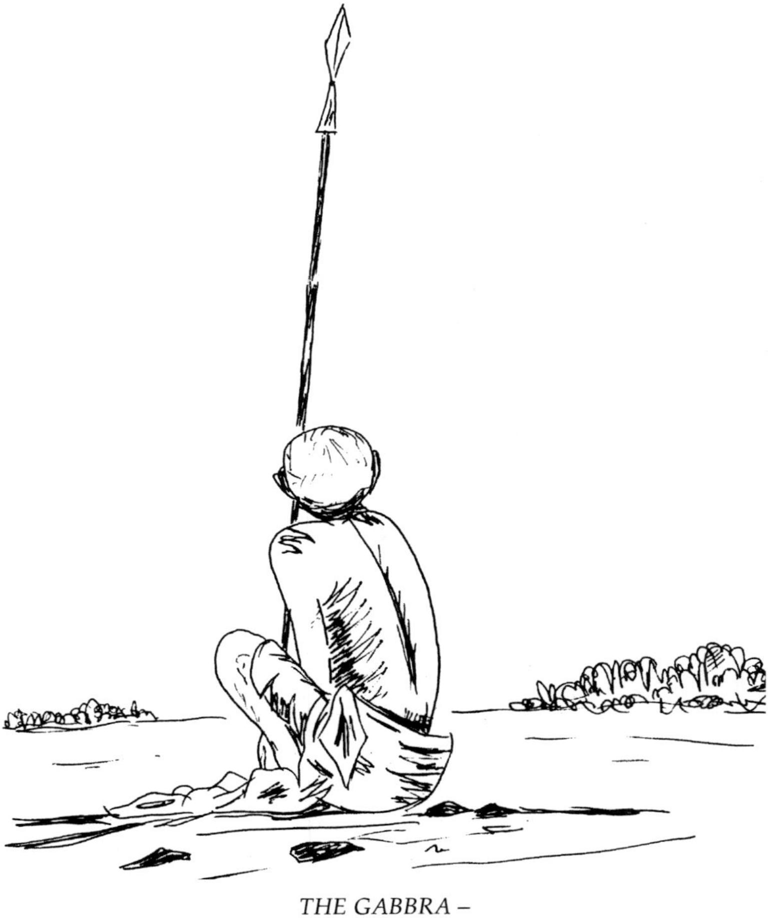

THE GABBRA –
PATIENTLY WATCHING HIS CAMELS AT A WATERING HOLE

The Gabbra along with the Turkana, Pokot, Samburu and Rendille are referred to as the Shepherds of the desert. The Gabbra live in a dwelling which is akin to a tent and their territory extends to the west of Lake Turkana and towards Marsabit. When conditions are unfavourable they simply take their house down, pack it onto the back of their camel and move on to better conditions. More and more of them however are becoming communal and sedentary, living around water holes as we witnessed in Kalacha. here they water their animals, grow vegetables and sugar cane. The Gabbra tribesmen we travelled with were usually easy to get on with and certainly very keen to ask for medical help.

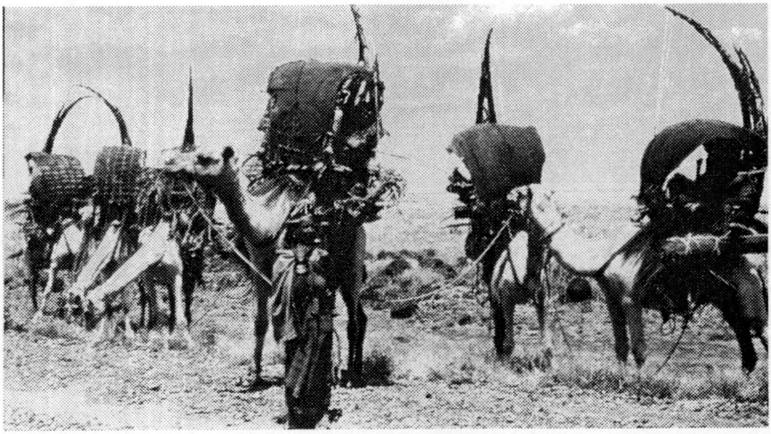

THE GABBRA ON THE MOVE

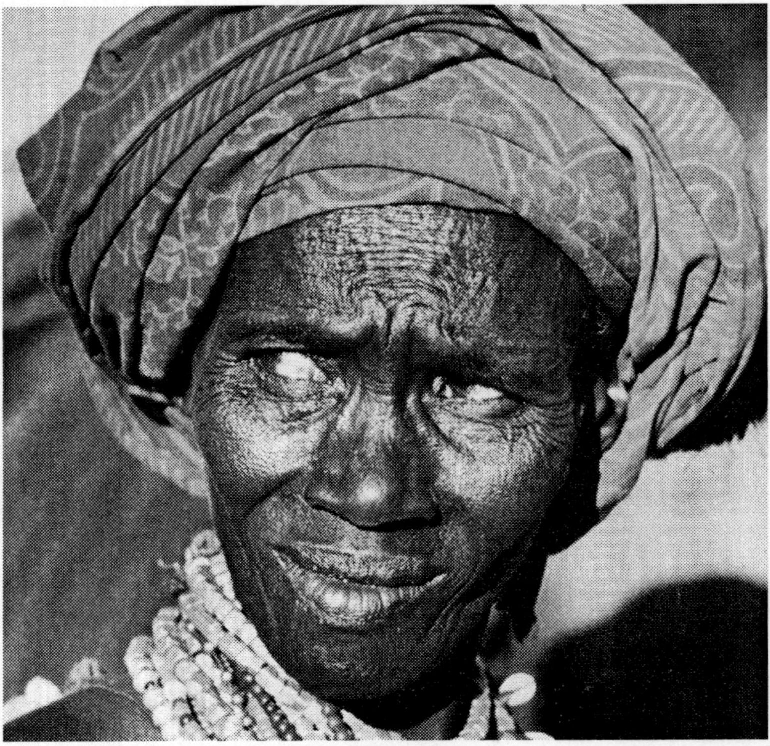

A WIDOW – After the rite called Negressa *(she has had her head shaved) and will be allowed to let her hair grow again*

we were proudly shown around by the head man of the village. He also showed us the school they had built and discussed with Peter the problems they had with the education of their children. On our return to the camp Peter told us he had arranged for the head man to visit our camp the next day and informed us that he felt we should give some donation towards the upkeep of the school and help with their problems. We all readily agreed. The next day he arrived with other elders of the tribe and he was also accompanied by his daughter. We presented them with money to buy books and writing materials and the chief's daughter, who was at university in Nairobi, agreed to do the purchasing. Once again, as on previous expeditions I have been on with Peter, the relationship between ourselves and the local people was of a very high standard.

The Gabbra belong culturally to the family of the Galla and

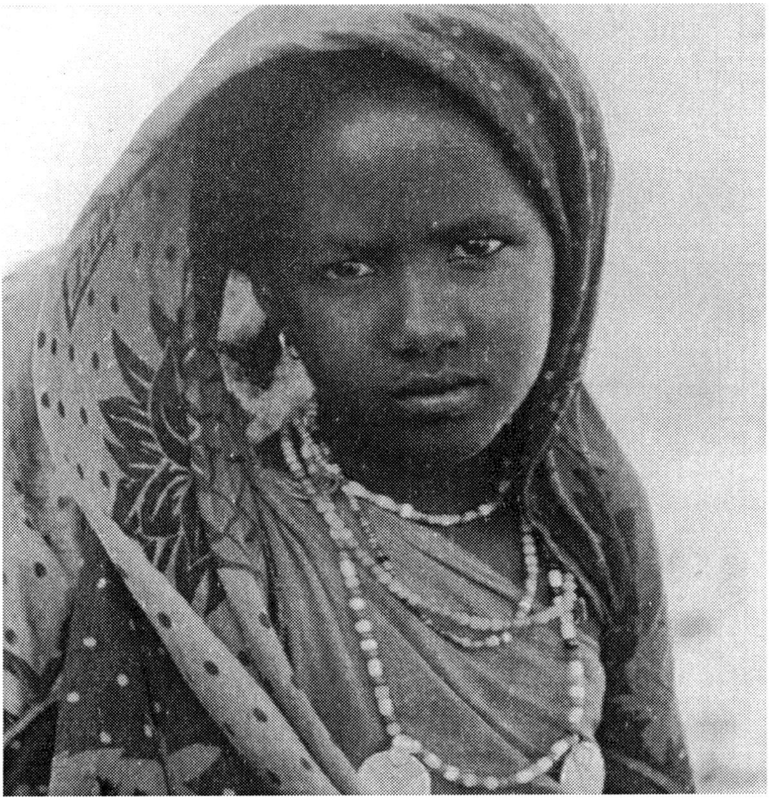

YOUNG GABBRA GIRL

number about 25,000. The Galla came originally from the more northern part of Africa. The Gabbra territory covers roughly 35,000 square miles, east of Lake Turkana in the district of Marsabit. It is an area which in the dry season gives the impression of boundless, deserted and inhospitable expanses of stones, broken in places by patches of dried grass and thorny shrub turning into absolute desert. In the wet season, however, the plains are all green, full of flowers an washed by tumultuous and flooding rivers.

The Gabbra are nomads and herdsmen of camels and cattle and are described as being the shepherds of the desert. Their culture can only be understood really as an ability to survive in extremely adverse conditions and with a social organisation well adapted to a nomad way of life. They tend to be tall and thin and dress simply. The men wear white shamahs and women dresses of attractive colours. They live in dwellings made of skins and vegetable matter which resembles something between a hut and a tent. These dwellings are resistant to strong winds and are adapted to their frequent migrations. If conditions become difficult they simply take it down, put it on the back of their camels and go somewhere else, so they can find water for their camels, sheep and goats.

They tend to have one wife only although polygamy is accepted. The live in small villages of about ten to fifteen families. Each village is ruled by an elder who is referred to as the father of the village. The elders meet and settle questions related to grazing areas, migrations and disputes amongst the tribe. The animals are owned by the head of the family while the land belongs to the tribe.

The Gabbra know the solar year after a system of their own but do not count the years of man as we do. They have adapted a system referred to as the Gadda system and this is a set of stages or age-set. Every seven years there is a general graduation of all the people. With circumcision they enter the first stage, then the warrior stage, the junior elder stage and finally the senior. Some become the Abba-Olla who is the father of the village. Pastoral life and home craft persist as the basic activities for both men and women. With camels, heads of cattle, goats and sheep all the male population give their time to the care of the herds, construction of paddocks, watering, milking, butchering and tanning of hides. The married women busy themselves providing food and looking after their children as well as practising textiles and woodcraft.

Rain and peace are the two basic values of the Gabbra society. What a refreshing attitude compared to ours in the west, where wars are constant and the bank balance seems to take priority. The Gabbra who crave for peace within the tribe may become aggressive with surrounding tribes if threatened, with the exception of the Boran and the Rendille tribes with whom they have formed an understanding. Their traditional enemies are the Samburu and the Shanghilla. If one of the enemy is killed in battle the warrior receives glory within the tribe. He is adorned with a large ivory ring on his arm and is exalted by everybody.

Hunting dangerous animals - the lion or rhino - is practised as a form of strength and courage within the tribe and again women will celebrate the brave warrior with songs and dances and reward him with ostrich feathers and necklaces.

It was interesting to watch and observe the ways of life that the Gabbra pursued in Kalacha. This was evidence of a more modern society; they had a runway in the village, a school, a clinic run by a nurse but there was ample evidence that for some of them life had not changed for centuries. They still lived a primitive form of life and this was sharply contrasted by the sudden appearance of a light aircraft on the runway. I wondered how soon it would be before their way of life was eroded by modern-day man. I suppose you cannot remain totally isolated in this modern world any more. This idea left me with a feeling of sadness and regret.

We met up with our trucks again in Kalacha, packed all our gear aboard and set off again on our journey. We said good-bye to the chief and the elders and set off in the direction of North Horr and then to the shores of Lake Turkana, The Jade sea, the home of the Turkana tribe and the El Molo. Our visit there would be short and then we would head south again towards Nairobi.

The next day after travelling across the Chalbi desert we arrived at North Horr where we met the priest in charge of the mission there. An enormous unfinished church dominated the mission grounds; it left me feeling uneasy when I realised how much money must have been spent on it and I looked around at the homes and standard of living of the local tribes. Perhaps the money could have been used more wisely. Having said that, there was a school nearby full of the noise and laughter of children. I was introduced to the nurse in charge of the clinic, left some of the medical gear I could spare and we then left towards Loiyangalani on the eastern shores of the lake, arriving in the early afternoon. We looked around the village for somewhere to

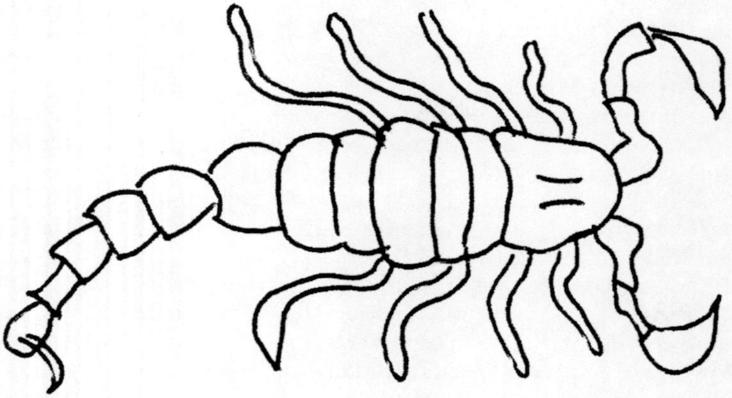

SCORPIONS: ANDROCTONUS AENAS
About 3″ – 4″ long and common in Northern Kenya

Scorpions are active at night and spend the day in shelter, as do many other desert animals. They use their claws to catch their prey and then kill it using its poison stored in the tail. Fatal cases are unusual but the problem may be different in young children. Most stings although not life threatening are very painful and best dealt with by injecting local anaesthetic at the site of the bite. As in most aspects of expedition medicine prevention is better than cure. Before setting up camp look for scorpion holes and dig them out. Be careful collecting wood and always inspect your boots before putting them on. It is a good idea on expeditions in the desert to take with you a pillow case and at night put your clothes and boots in it and then use it as a pillow. Any member walking around in bare feet is likely to incur the wrath of the expidition doctor. During the day they are not difficult to find by kicking over a large stone where they rest in the heat of the day – but are best left alone. It is not difficult to find trouble in a desert – so do not go looking for it.

camp but decided to head further south and spend the night along the shores of the lake. It was here that we camped and saw the Turkana fishing in the lake. Apart from fishing they hunt both crocodile and hippos from the shore rushing into the water with nets and spears. Not an occupation for the faint-hearted.! They became aggressive as we approached them and taking photographs was done at the risk of life and limb. The gentle colours as evening came were unforgettable - it must have been a water-colour artist's paradise. The sun set over the lake and we sat in rows to watch the sun go down. It was almost like being at the cinema but the screen was the horizon. After the sun had set we set about retiring for the night and it was then that one of the girls let out a scream. Scorpions, dozens of scorpions, big ones, little ones and whole families of scorpions. I then realised what people meant when they said the desert comes to life at night. They scurried and scuttled around in the camp site - it was like the organisation of the Scorpion Grand National! We built up the fire, moved our camp beds even closer and, finally, after calming things down, went to sleep.

Early the next day before we set off for Nairobi Peter gave a brief talk to the expedition as it was now drawing to a close. I remember thinking how lucky we had been from a medical point of view. I had dealt with the usual cuts and bruises, the unexplained abdominal pain, comforted and calmed down the nervous, attended to several of the Gabbra but nothing dramatic or serious had happened. Little did I know what the day after would bring as we approached Nairobi. Never again will I count my blessings until I reach home, sweet home.

Our next destination was Maralal where we spent the night, but on our way we stopped off at South Horr. Here I visited a mission hospital run by Italian nuns. I left more of my medical equipment with the nurses. You must wonder if I had enough medical gear to look after the expedition but I always carry too much, with the idea in mind of leaving some at the various places I visit.

APPENDICITIS AND TROUBLE

The next day, having had a good night's sleep and having filled our stomachs on goat's meat and vegetables, we set off on the final leg of our journey, hoping to arrive in Nairobi late in the afternoon. On our way we were to stop off and admire the view at Thomsons Falls. As we drew close one of the young scouts complained of abdominal pain and with difficulty I examined him in the back of the truck. He was tender in the lower right hand part of his abdomen but it was nothing too serious. I decided to get to Thomsons Falls and examine him again, suspecting he might have had appendicitis. An hour later we arrived and by this time there was no doubt about the diagnosis. The view of the falls was spectacular but as I examined him I realised that the sooner we arrived in Nairobi the better and after giving him some antibiotics and something to relieve his pain we set off. The first problem we had was a puncture in the truck but after an hour's delay we started off once again. Appendicitis in this country is not pleasant but being bumped about in a truck with peritonitis certainly isn't. He rapidly became ill with pain and the infection proceeded at a brisk pace. I gave him further sedation and put up a drip. We were still about four hours' away from Nairobi and I decided he had had enough so we tried to contact the Flying Doctor service. To do this you had to find a runway and a telephone, neither of which we could locate, so in the end we abandoned the idea and made a dash to Nairobi. I will never forget that journey and I am sure the young scout will not either. Every bump caused him further pain and with him heavily sedated and wedged between myself and the side of the truck we continued the horrendous journey. We finally arrived at the hospital in Nairobi much later than expected, collected a trolley from the casualty department and wheeled him in. I was met by a beaming casualty sister and when I told her where we had travelled from I do not think she believed me. The young lad was examined by an Asian doctor who had just finished working in Dundee and he agreed with the diagnosis. About an hour later the surgeon arrived and made arrangements for the patient to be operated on. He also assured me there was no risk of the Aids infection and left. By this time I was absolutely exhausted and as the scout fell asleep on the trolley, I fell asleep on a bench in the corridor. The casualty sister woke us, beaming at us. 'You are going to the theatre' she said to the scout 'and you, doctor, are coming with me.' They took him away and I followed the sister into the nurses rest room where she offered me a cup of tea and a biscuit. I drank the tea quickly and then ate my way through the packet of biscuits. She laughed and poured me more tea and then I fell asleep again. About an hour later I was told I was wanted on the phone and spoke to the surgeon who had successfully removed the boy's appendix. He assured me the lad was fine and had been taken to the ward. The patients in the hospital had a choice of treatment and I just marked everything private and handed the form back to them. He would have a private room , private nurse and private everything if it was available. I really felt he deserved the best they had to offer. I wandered up to the ward after thanking the casualty sister, who was still beaming and found him peacefully sleeping in bed. I was very jealous! It had been a long day; we had started at dawn and it was now after ten o'clock at night.

I had been in his room about ten minutes when there was a knock on the door and in walked Peter with two of the leaders. I related to him the events of the day and after finally checking the scout was alright and speaking to the night sister on duty we left back towards Hillcrest School. There there was a change of clothes after a shower, some food and alcohol and I collapsed on my camp bed. Sleep was not long coming that night! The care and treatment he received in the hospital was of the highest order. They had been courteous and efficient and over the next few days we visited him regularly. He eventually returned home with us fit and well and recovered from his ordeal.

CORPORAL DAVID

The tale of the Kenyan expedition would not be complete without mentioning Corporal David. He was a black African, built like a brick wall and in charge of the young African scouts who joined us on our trek. He was a member of the GSU - the general service unit - a branch of the Kenyan police. These policemen were trained by the SAS. Corporal David was a professional man of the highest order and he kept us enthralled at night by recounting his exploits.

On the Ethiopian-Kenyan border guerillas come from the north with the intent of killing elephant for their ivory and generally grabbing or stealing whatever they can and they don't mind how they do it. There is a spotter plane that flies just south of the border in Kenya and is on the lookout for bandits coming from the north. If they are spotted a message is relayed to base and two helicopter gun ships take off in search of them. Their position is marked by a flare. The helicopters swoop down straffing with automatic gunfire and having repeated this exercise they land. No prisoners are taken now as the Kenyan police lost several personnel by a more gentle approach of questioning and persuasion; needless to say, this activity has declined rapidly but despite this vigilance the fate of the poor elephant still hangs in the balance. Corporal David was in charge of one of these helicopters.

His fitness was unbelievable. At a camp site south of Isiolo in central Kenya he was noticed one evening by his absence. He returned some three hours later as we chatted by the fire late at night. He appeared from the darkness, covered in sweat and grinning from ear to ear. He had apparently run to Isiolo and then back. He was obviously aware of the dangers of such a trip but had not been deterred. Not like some of us I could name!

His map reading was outstanding. When the truck had broken down because of a broken axle (we were some three miles from Karabara) he decided to find the village even though it was late evening to try and summon help. Again he was undeterred and vanished into the night. He was dressed in his field kit, two knives on his belt and a piece of rope. Impressed, I stood in amazement at this man even more as we had heard there were lion in the near vicinity. True to form he returned after a couple of hours and on his return presented me with a porcupine quill he had found!

My younger daughter who accompanied me on the trip was in awe and admiration for such a man as we all were - but found it difficult to marry the kindness and concern he showed us with the fact that David was a trained killer.

I remember sitting by the fire on our first night in the bush listening to him deliver a lecture on survival in the bush. He warned about its dangers, enthused about its beauty and explained to us we were honoured to be in such a remote and wild place. He finished by saying that we should leave it as we found it. All camp sites had to be kept tidy and the environment protected.

The care he showed us was outstanding. If anyone was upset or frightened he would reassure them - if we wanted wood for the fire he would find it. At first he insisted on staying awake all night to protect us. Every time I saw this man I saw another facet of his character.

So who was Corporal David? He was a policeman trained in self-defence and survival; he was kind and gentle but I was left in no doubt if there was trouble I would be much relieved if he were near at hand! He was good-looking and had an eye for the girls as we witnessed in the hospital in Nairobi. When we were concerned about our patient, Corporal David was chatting up the local nurses! He was a conservationist and above all easy to approach and open in sharing his thoughts and problems. I spent several hours talking to him and our relationship became a good one - each respecting the other and listening to each other's point of view.

It has never failed to amaze me on my journeys how different people exhibit the cornerstones of human behaviour: caring, sharing and listening, and how a sense of humour can rapidly advance a relationship. Corporal David was a fine example of this and I learned much from this remarkable Kenyan. I have met him on four occasions now and look forward to our next meeting.

THE WELSH NURSE AND MEASLES

Kalacha is a stable Gabbra community in the Northern Frontier District of Kenya and like most stable tribal settlements has its own mission clinic. The clinic here was run by a jovial, somewhat overweight Welsh nurse. I spent one afternoon going through her medical equipment with her and leaving what medical gear I could. I replaced and added what I could spare. The clinic was set back from the runway and near the water mill. There was a veranda and inside I found three rooms. A kitchen in some state of disarray, a small bed room which was not much better and a store room containing food, bedding and some dressing packs for her to use on her visits. Most of her time was spent visiting the Gabbra settlements in the area. She was a trained midwife and told several hair-raising stories about her work in that remote area. The nearest hospital was at Marsabit some six hours away. She worked alone with little or no back-up team. After we had finished sorting her medical gear out we sat chatting outside sitting on the veranda.

'The major cause of death in children around here,' she started, 'is measles and several children die each year, but I think I have cracked it,' she went on with a great beaming smile on her face. For years she had been trying to persuade the elders of the tribes to immunise their children against this killer disease but they had all stubbornly refused. One day in an outlying village she managed to persuade one of the elders to allow her to carry out a limited immunisation course. Having done this, the word spread and several other villages also wished to take part in the programme. This she refused to do. The next year brought its inevitable outbreak and some children died of measles, but not one single one died in the small village she had immunised. She then carried out one of the most successful immunisation programmes ever undertaken; virtually every child in her district was successfully immunised and there has not been a single death since. 'What about that,' she commented with a grin on her face from ear to ear.

'Brilliant' I replied 'absolutely brilliant.' In that one exercise she accomplished more than most of us could hope to do in a lifetime.

'I will put the kettle on,' she said as she stood up and headed for the kitchen. 'No you will not' I replied, reaching into my rucksack and pulling out a water bottle half full of brandy. 'We will drink to your success with this.' She soon returned with two glasses and we toasted her accomplishment courtesy of a bottle of Napoleon brandy. 'This is purely medicinal,' I commented, with a smile on my face.

The most successful things in life and medicine are usually the most simple and this was a good example. With patience and determination that Welsh nurse had planned and persisted with her purpose. When things looked bad she never gave up and then devised a simple plan, with some cunning, to enable her to complete her mission. The reward were beyond her wildest dreams. Healthier kids and no measles. Life appears to be so much more simple in this country. We are given measles protection as a routine measure and certainly in twenty years of work in general practice I have never seen a death attributed to measles. What a comparison!

Before we left Kalacha I went to say my good-byes to her. She was standing on the veranda and, as usual, her face was covered by her delightful smile. She said she was grateful for the drugs and dressings I had given her and I gave her a big hug before I left. That was yet another person I will never forget on my travels as an expedition doctor.

SOUTH HORR AND THE ITALIAN NUNS

At South Horr in northern Kenya is a small, well run mission hospital. It is run by Italian nuns who man it twenty-four hours a day. This is Samburu country and it was here that we stopped, having left Lake Turkana in the north on our way back to Nairobi.

It was a glorious day as we drew up outside the mission hospital at about midday. Outside sitting on benches was a line of local people waiting to be seen. I was introduced to the sister in charge, a middle-aged, friendly, smiling nun called Marta Polo. After a few pleasantries she invited us into the clinic where she asked me to see a screaming two-year-old with a large umbilical hernia who had been vomiting. I think she thought the hernia was obstructing the bowel and that was why the child was vomiting, but it also had diarrhoea and I came to the conclusion that if we could stop the child crying the hernia would reduce itself. After the skilled attention of another nun the child stopped crying and the hernia reduced itself. 'I think the child will be alright,' I said 'but keep it here for a day or two until the gastroenteritis settles.' She smiled and then her face changed. 'We have a different problem here' she said and I followed her into the adjoining cubicle.

On a chair sat a young Samburu mother with a child held in her arms. I bent down to attend to the child and very quickly realised that it was severely anaemic in heart failure and obviously dying. I stood up and looked at sister Marta Polo and walked away from the mother and child. 'The child is dying,' I whispered to her, 'it probably has cerebral malaria but if we don't take it with us to Nairobi it will certainly die.' 'At least if we take the child it may stand a chance.' The nun turned to the cubicle and told the mother our intentions. The mother would not let her child go as her husband had left her and there was nobody to look after the other children. 'Tell her we will take the family with us,' I replied and once again she disappeared into the cubicle. She re-emerged two minutes later. 'She will not let her child go as there is nobody to feed the goats!' she stated. That was it as far as I was concerned - 'bloody hell, sister' I exploded. 'This is crazy.' She put her hand on my forearm and, looking me in the face, said, 'this is Africa doctor, and it is not your fault.' She repeated this twice to me as she must have seen the look of astonishment on my face. I suddenly felt humble and somewhat stupid and apologised for my outburst.

The sister walked over to the other side of the clinic and spoke softly to another nun who left the room only to emerge five minutes later with a bowl of fruit. The mother with her baby, the two nuns and I stood in the cubicle and ate some of the fruit. I remember thinking - "who was supposed to be treating who!"

There was nothing else I could do and soon we left the nuns with a distinct feeling of being totally and utterly useless. 'Good-bye and thank you,' I said to the sister. 'I have learned a lot today about the problems you face. I just wish I could have done more.' She gave me an understanding look and we left in the direction of Nairobi. Once, on our journey I nudged Peter in the ribs. 'I am coming back here,' I said determinedly. He said nothing and we continued our journey in silence.

It is amazing the different priorities and problems that parents have in the world. Here was a mother with a dying child in her arms and she would not let it go. As I reflected on the incident I realised that the mother's responsibility was to the family as a whole and not just the child. She must have been obviously more devastated than I was. It was easy to criticise and become angry but it certainly wasn't your position to do so. Life can be very hard in Africa - very hard indeed.

This was the second time I had encountered a mother with a dying child who had refused to let me try and help. You are left with an empty feeling and a determination to come back and try to do more. It is difficult also when you return home and treat the patients with whom you can find little the matter. It certainly leaves you very frustrated and takes some coming to terms with. Perhaps I should leave general practice in England and go and work out there but I have a feeling the frustrations would only continue. This situation really set my mind buzzing. If I could reach these places why couldn't medical care? The ramifications of that are endless - politicians, money and so on. So I had better stay where I am, but even that still sounds defeatist.

DOCTORS THINK THEY ARE CLEVER DEVILS

It must have been about eight o'clock in the evening. We were camping in the bush in northern Kenya and the scene was dominated by Mount Feroli. One of the Gabbra camel herders came into the camp to ask if one of the doctors would come and attend to one of the elders of the tribe who was travelling with them. They were camping about a hundred yards away in a dried-out river bed. I struggled through the darkness to find my patient lying down with the other Gabbra crowded around him. They were obviously very concerned about him. I knelt down and tried to find out what was the matter. The only information I could elicit was that he appeared to be in a coma and barely rousable. I examined him as best I could but was still none the wiser. I diagnosed cerebral malaria as the commonest cause of these symptoms and gave him some tablets. Well, it didn't seem a bad diagnosis at the time. I reached into my friendly medical rucksack and gave him some white tablets of quinine and more yellow tablets of oxytetracycline. I left enough therapy for the next three days. They managed to lift his head and after struggling we put them in his mouth. I left instructions that if he worsened in the night to call me. I did not know what I would do but at least I could think of something! I wandered back to our camp with Peter in the dark. 'I have not a clue what that was

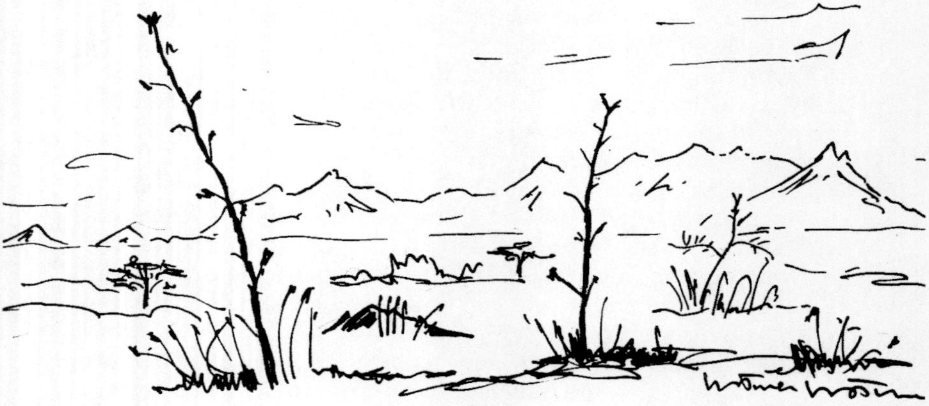

FEROLI RANGE

about,' I remarked. 'He certainly looked ill but did not appear to be dying.' I was left with a distinct feeling of unease. Before I went to sleep that night it was still on my mind. 'If he dies we've had it,' I commented to Peter before we dropped off to sleep. I did not sleep much that night and wondered what the next day would bring.

In the morning I was amazed to see him loading gear on the camels as if nothing had happened the night before and he kept nodding his head at me and smiling. In appreciation of my efforts to help him, or so I thought. I watched him on and off during the day and there was no doubt he had made a full recovery. I felt quite pleased with my previous night's endeavours.

I was relating this story to the Welsh nurse who worked in the mission hospital in Kalacha and a great smile appeared on her face. I finished by saying that I had never seen cerebral malaria before but the man had responded quickly to the treatment. 'You have been fooled,' she laughed, 'white and yellow tablets fetch a high price around here.' She laughed even louder. 'He was not nodding his head in appreciation. He was working out how much money he would make and will have probably pocketed the proceeds!' I felt a complete and utter fool and must have looked somewhat dejected. She tapped my leg and roared her head off and soon we were both laughing together.

Life as an expedition doctor can certainly have it's problems and this was no exception. You think you know it all but it does you no harm to be brought back to earth with a bump! I suppose one of the secrets is to let as few people as possible know what happened and I am not quite sure why I'm relating this story to you but I hope it makes you laugh as much as it did the Welsh nurse. I had been completely taken in by the 'sick' man and obviously was not the clever devil I thought I was! Not only had he fooled me but had also made a profit into the bargain - the swine!

JASPER AND HIS CAMELS

About twenty-five kilometres north of Rumaruti travelling along dirt roads you come across an eight-foot high stone on the left-hand side of the road. On it in fading white paint are painted the initials J.E. This marks the turn-off to the farm of Jasper Evans, one of the last white hunters in northern Kenya. Rumaruti is on the road between Thomson Falls and Maralal. This is Samburu country. Jasper Evans has lived here all his life except for a short spell in the Royal Navy. He lives here with his wife Jill and farms an area of some 30,000 acres surrounded by eighty miles of fencing. On this land he looks after and manages cattle, goats and sheep, but undoubtedly his great love is camels. Scattered over his farm are African villages comprising settlement of about ten to twenty mud huts with grass roofs. In each of these villages is a head man responsible for maintaining discipline and looking after his stock.

Early one morning at about seven o'clock I found myself sitting in the back of his land-rover travelling to one of these villages. One of his head men had been caught stealing goats and Jasper was on his way to sort the problem out. Once we arrived and jumped out of the land-rover there was no doubt as to who was in control. The offending man was duly summoned and received a piece of Jasper's mind. The look on his crest-fallen face told the story. The problem was quickly resolved as Jasper took his rifle from him with the instruction that he would return in a few days and give the rifle back providing he returned the goats.

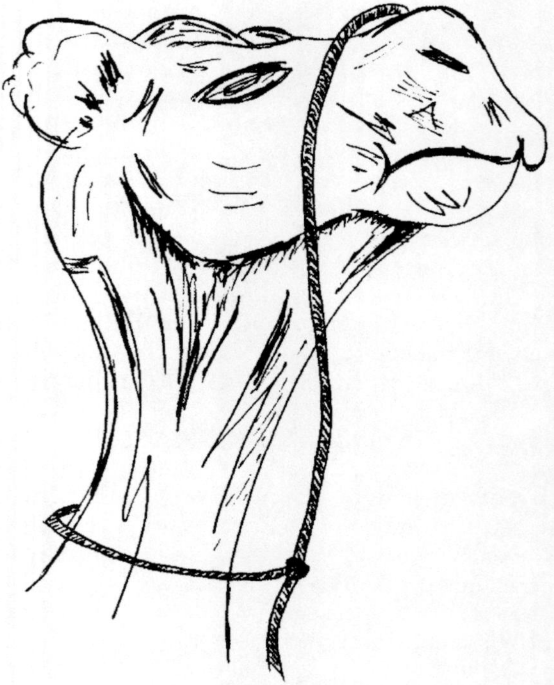

THE CAMEL
– Supebly Adapted to Desert Life

On the way back to the farm we passed a small herd of camels - there were about thirty all together grazing in the bush. 'Camels are fantastic and beautiful creatures' he said, and with that he slammed on the breaks and leaped out of his vehicle in their direction. 'Come on' he said 'come and meet them.' He walked into the middle of the herd and stroked and patted them. Here was a man at peace with his environment. Never have I witnessed such a scene of care and love between and man and beast. He obviously felt great affection for these ships of the desert. Younger camels nuzzled at this neck and the whole scene was one of peace and tranquillity - man at peace with his beloved camels. At first we followed with trepidation and doubt but these fears were soon resolved as soon we were also patting and stroking these magnificent animals. 'After one desert trip, one of my camels drank 104 litres of water' he said with pride. I estimated that to be about a dustbin full! There is a down side to camels, as I found out; they make the most disgusting noises and can be somewhat temperamental. Jasper Evans must be one of the world's experts in camel management and it was both a privilege and a pleasure to be in the company of this remarkable man.

Soon we were back on his land-rover travelling back to the farm. It was a hair-raising journey as we bumped and sped along at great speed along desert tracks. We arrived back just in time for breakfast - porridge, bacon and toast, all washed down with delicious Kenyan coffee.

After breakfast we walked slowly back to the garden at the back of the farm. 'Doctor,' said Jasper, 'one of my camels has a bad cut in it's mouth and I'm very worried about it - would you come and have a look at it?' 'Certainly,' I said, grabbing my medical bag and following him to a small fenced off area at the rear of the farm. Here we found five Africans leading a camel who I assumed correctly was the patient. 'Hang on,' he said 'we'll hobble the camel so you can have a look.' With that the camel was soon tied up, not unlike a Christmas turkey, all four legs tied up with the Africans' help. Three of them sat on the camels side, one wrapping himself around the camel's neck and the last gripping the camel by it's upper lip and holding it's head.

Once I had cleaned the camel's mouth with the help of a bowl of water I could see there was a large laceration from the lower dental margin extending into the floor of the camel's mouth. It was bleeding quite heavily. It was apparent to me that it would be difficult to stitch together as there was little tissue by the lower dental margin. I was hesitant at first but there was no doubt Jasper wanted me to have a go. I stitched the upper part of the wound with difficulty, the lower flap posing no problems. As I drew the suture material together, the catgut easily pulled out of the upper part of the wound. 'I will have another go' I said and this time I pushed the needle deeper into the camel's mouth. The result was disaster as the unfortunate beast reacted violently. The Africans sitting on its flanks were thrown off; the one hanging on to its neck went flying backwards and the one holding its upper lip was tossed over the camel's head and sent me flying backwards! I found myself lying on my back, my arms outstretched and in my right hand was a very bent suturing needle. Jasper Evans with his hands on his hips was roaring with laughter! 'I bet this is a little different to general practice in Accrington.' he exploded and continued in convulsions of laughter. I soon picked myself up and in a short time I was peering once more into the camel's mouth. Once again I washed the wound but the bleeding continued. 'Iodine' I shouted, 'iodine, there is a bottle of iodine in the kitchen.' With that, Jasper set off in the direction of the farm. He soon returned with his trophy. Carefully we painted the wound with iodine, the bleeding stopped and Jasper seemed well pleased with my efforts. 'I think the camel will be OK,' I said, 'the laceration will not stop the camel feeding or drinking but I suggest you repeat this over the next few days on a daily basis to prevent the wound becoming infected.'

I collected what was left of my equipment together, the camel was released into another fenced off area and proceeded at a brisk trot. As Jasper and I wandered back to the farm he put his hand on my shoulder. 'Ever thought of becoming a vet?' he smiled at me. When I thought of budget holding, cash flow and target payments, I must admit I became very tempted!

What a fabulous start to the day it had been. Caring, sorting a difficult problem out and being able to help a man so keen to make sure his camels had the best of attention. The whole experience had given me an intense feeling of satisfaction, accompanied by a sore backside!

THE ULCERATED FOOT AND THE CHEETAH'S TOOTH

As you leave Rumaruti in Northern Kenya on the way to Maralal the tarmac road finishes and the track becomes dirt consisting of sand, stones and rubble with frequent potholes as it winds its way through the semi-scrub desert. After being shaken like a rag

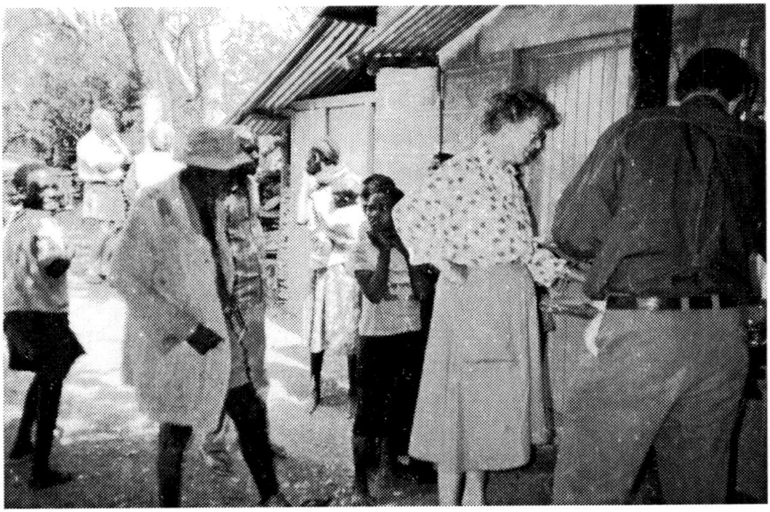

↑ *The young boy with the ulcerated foot*

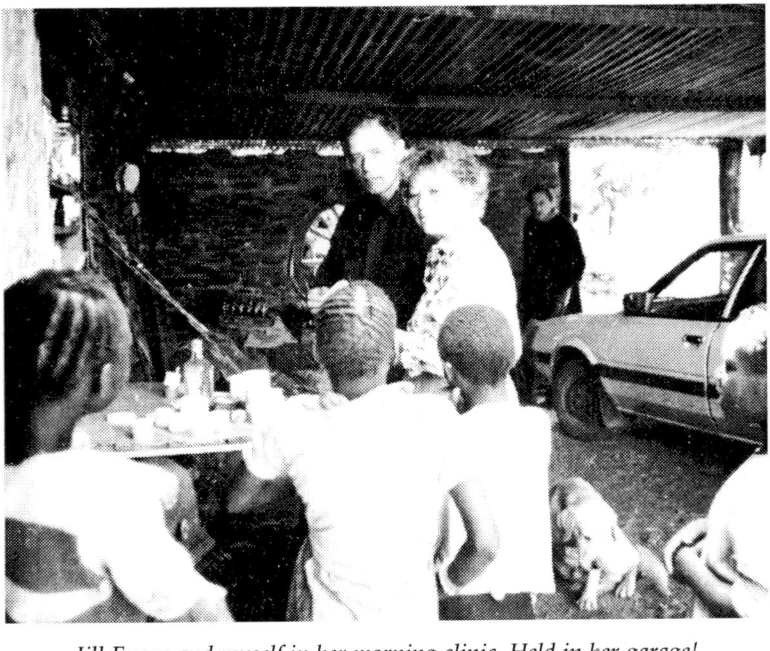

Jill Evans and myself in her morning clinic. Held in her garage!

doll in a land-rover for about twenty-five kilometres you arrive at the entrance to the farm of Jasper Evans on the left-hand side of the track. After turning for about a hundred yards you arrive at the garage which marks the entrance to the farmhouse. It is a double-built wooden garage in a somewhat sorry state of repair. It was here that I found myself one bright and sunny morning in February.

At the entrance to the rear of the garage is a large cupboard containing medicine bottles, dressings and antibiotic powders. Standing in front of this and facing a queue of local Samburu was Jill Evans carrying out her morning surgery. One child of about two years, accompanied by his mum, had a cough fever and vomiting. Jill was giving him cough medicine and vitamin tablets. 'They love the tablets,' she said 'they are a bright colour but I don't know if they do any good.' 'Sure they do,' I said, 'just as long as they think they are then it must be doing them good.' The next in the queue was an elderly man leaning on his stick complaining of backache. 'I think he's strained his back,' she said. 'Ask him about his waterworks,' I said. 'Has he trouble passing urine and does it hurt or is there blood in his urine?' The answer was that, although water was difficult to pass and it was often painful, there was no blood. I reached into my rucksack and asked her to give him some antibiotics with the suggestion that she should see him in a couple of days to see if he had improved. 'If he's no better then you are probably right.' But I did wonder about his prostate gland and the possibility of a kidney infection.

The next patient to present himself was a young boy of about eight years with bright white eyes shining out of his black smiling face. He sat on the ground and lifted up his foot to reveal a large healing ulcer on its dorsal aspect. It was obviously healing. 'I am impressed,' I said, 'you really have done well here.' Although he was obviously pleased with his foot the ulcer was sloughing and still painful. 'Honey,' I exclaimed 'honey!' I had seen a jar in the kitchen. 'Put some honey on the wound, it will help it to heal.' With that Jill Evans shot off in the direction of the farm only to return in two minutes clasping a jar of wild honey. She expertly re-dressed the foot and with an even larger smile on his face the young patient expressed his satisfaction. All three of us were suitably pleased and she agreed to see him in a couple of days. I felt great admiration for this nurse working in such conditions and in such a devoted way. It is amazing what you can do when you have to improvise! Soon the queue dwindled - more coughs and colds and more cough linctus and vitamin tablets and more satisfied patients. I had really enjoyed my morning with her; certainly a change from general practice in Lancashire.

In the rear of the garage sitting on a shelf was a row of four lion skulls and I saw Peter looking intently at them. 'One of these would be fabulous for my son to take to school,' he said. 'What facts they could learn from one of these. 'Ask Jasper if you can have one,' I suggested, 'I'm sure he could sort something out for you.'

True to form in about two minutes Peter and I were travelling in the front of Jasper's land-rover heading to a local village. 'I would like to keep those,' he remarked, but there should be one in the village to which we are heading. After about fifteen minutes we drew up outside a small community of about twelve mud and thatched huts and in the middle of these stood a wooden hut with a locked door. Jasper summoned the head man who soon appeared clutching a bunch of keys and after struggling with the lock opened the door. Inside on shelves were stacks of animal skins, mainly camel, but on the floor scattered under the shelves were the skulls of various animals. The head man was being helped by several young boys eagerly searching out a lion's skull but all to no avail. Jasper Evans was furious. 'They have stolen them!' he exploded, 'and sold them or made them into necklaces using the teeth as beads.' It was obvious that Peter was to be let down. 'Sorry,' repeated Jasper, still fuming about the whole incident.

As I was about to step into the land-rover I was aware of a young boy standing behind me with his hands clasped behind his back and I quickly recognised the gleaming smile on his face. It was the boy with the ulcer on his foot I had seen in the clinic earlier that morning. 'Hello,' I said cheerfully and went to meet him and put my hands on his face. I pointed to his foot and smiled, reassured him and gave him a hug. In a flash his hands appeared from behind his back and he proudly presented me with a cheetah's skull which he placed in my hands. 'Thank you,' I said and stuffed it up my jumper. As we drove off I waved back at him until he disappeared from view.

Back at the garage I revealed my prize to Peter. On closer inspection the skull was badly damaged but in the top jaw were two gleaming white teeth. 'What about one of these for your sons to take to school?' I remarked intensely. 'Brilliant,' he said, 'absolutely brilliant.' And soon we prized them from the cheetah's skull. One tooth went into his back pocket and the other into mine. As we passed the row of lions skulls at the back of the garage I carefully placed the cheetah's skull with those of the lions.

What a fabulous day I had experienced. I had helped Jill Evans with her clinic but more than that had reached the heart of a young Samburu. In an incredible short time I had bonded with him and he with me. I have the tooth at home and I treasure it greatly. It had taught me so much. It taught me about people helping people but most of all it reminded me of the words of a Dutch distirct nurse who said to me when I first entered general practice. 'Remember doctor, that people will be with you as you are with them.'

THE NIGHT OF THE HAIRY CATERPILLARS

As we were eating dinner at about eight o'clock in the dining room at the farm of Jasper Evans in northern Kenya, I inadvertently looked up at the roof which had obviously been badly damaged. 'Young leopards,' he stated 'young leopards' repeated Jasper. 'We looked after them when their mother had been shot but we had to return them to the wild as they became so destructive.' He said it in such a matter-of-fact fashion. 'Leopards,' I said to myself, flipping leopards in your house!' I immediately thought of our cat peacefully sleeping on my knee at home. One of your distant relatives I remember laughing to myself.

The meal was brilliant, soup followed by zebra stew, fruit, cheese and biscuits. 'What are the sleeping arrangements?' Jasper quizzed his wife. All was apparently under control but there was a warning at the end. 'Hairy caterpillars' Jill remarked. 'There's a plague of them and you must inspect your beds before you get in them' she warned. 'If they crawl over you, they produce intense itching and pain accompanied by a red uncomfortable rash.'

After dinner we chatted in the lounge in front of an open log fire. Arranged on the chairs was an assortment of animal skins and a multitude of books adorned the bookcases. We discussed snake bites and their treatment, the problems of farming in northern Kenya but all too soon it was time for bed.

'Follow me,' exclaimed Jasper, as he leapt to his feet and Peter and I grabbed our rucksacks and sleeping bags and followed him into the night. He led us to the bottom of the garden to our sleeping quarters, the way illuminated by his torch. He unlocked the door, lit a lamp and with a hearty voice bade us goodnight and left.

We switched on our torches and inspected our home for the night. It was a stone-built dwelling with two beds in a small room and an adjoining bathroom. I teased Peter by jumping up and down waving my arms and pointing out the dangers of the hairy caterpillars. He was not impressed and with his torch diligently started searching the rooms looking earnestly into the corners. All of a sudden, the penny dropped - carpet vipers! In a similar situation two years before in northern Kenya in not dissimilar conditions we had found a carpet viper coiled up sleeping in the corner of a room. These snakes are lethal. The frivolity of the situation immediately became deadly serious. After a diligent and careful search we satisfied ourselves that we were alone. After a few minutes when we had unpacked our belongings I reminded him of the hairy caterpillars. We carefully peeled back each sheet and blanket and altogether collected four of the beasts. One in my bed and the other three in Peter's. We collected them with the assistance of my toothbrush and a piece of paper and dispatched them into the night.

Neither of us slept in the beds but crawled into our sleeping bags, zipped them up with only our faces peering into the dark. No carpet vipers, no more hairy caterpillars and a full stomach. Soon, after another exhausting day we both fell peacefully and safely asleep.

BOTSWANA

Botswana lies in southern Africa and is landlocked. It is surrounded by Zimbabwe in the east and South Africa in the south. Namibia forms the western border of the country and to the north and east lie Angola and Zambia. There is a thin stretch of land which is part of Namibia that runs from an east/westerly direction that separates northern Botswana from both Angola and Zambia in the north. This is called the Caprivi Strip. A journey along here is not at all pleasant; it is a long, hot and very dusty area.

Botswana itself is divided into four main regions. On the east side there is the Chobe and south of this there is Gabarone and the eastern corridor. To the west and the north lies the Okavango Delta system and to the south and the west lies the Kalahari Desert and this is by far the larger of the four distinct areas. It is a land of natural beauty and is seldom visited by the independent traveller. It is not a cheap place to visit, as it imports most of its goods from South Africa and the import tax is high. It still is very much dependent on support from South Africa. It is, however, a stable and a harmonious African country and became independent of British rule in 1964. Unlike Kenya, there is a multi-part democracy here.

At one time Botswana was regarded as one the poorest countries of Africa but it has been transformed largely by the discovery of diamonds, but also by the export of beef and the emerging tourist trade, into a prosperous country. It is now one of Africa's most rapidly developing economies. The capital of Botswana lies in Gabarone in the south and it is here that the president's office and administrative buildings lie. The city has been replanned and modernised but has little to endear itself to the visiting traveller. Compared with Zimbabwe or Kenya, Botswana is flat. It has been described by early explorers as miles and miles of bloody Africa. It is basically a shallow, sand-filled basin. Along the eastern corridor, however, lie a collection of small hills which form a watershed and it is here that most of the population live.

Travelling westwards, conditions are far less favourable and eventually give way to the harsh reality of the Kalahari Desert.

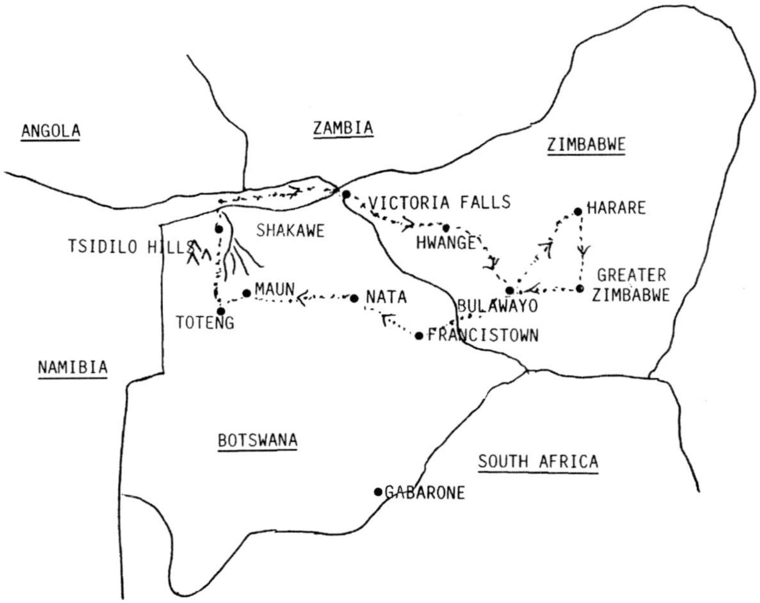

JOURNEY THROUGH ZIMBABWE AND BOTSWANA

This huge desert area has been largely populated by scrub, bush and open grasslands and forests. In the north, however, the country is different and is watered by the vast Okavango Delta system, which covers some fifteen thousand square miles and consists of channels, lakes and flood plains. It is here that wildlife abounds with hippos and crocodiles in the rivers and channels and a vast array of bird life. It is to here that the tourist trade has been attracted. The official language here is English and it is taught in the schools. However, other languages are spoken and Setswana is understood by a large majority of the population. This is a Bant language and brought to Botswana originally by the early tribes who settled here when they came many years ago from what is today South Africa.

The bushmen were the original inhabitants of Botswana, living in the Kalahari Desert. The poor bushmen seem to have been driven out from every other part of Africa and settled here where nobody else seemed to want to go.

The first white explorers of Botswana came from the south and they included the Dutch and also the British, but the most famous of them all was David Livingstone. He explored extensively in what is now Botswana and travelled north, eventually reaching the Zambesi River where he discovered the Victoria Falls which he named after his Queen. He also explored the land to the west, around the Okavango Delta system. His statue stands proud in the Victoria Falls park and this is a popular place to have your photograph taken.

The development of Botswana has been dramatic, especially over the last twenty years, and with their newly found wealth it must surely continue to grow. Education is flourishing and the medical care given to the local population is becoming of an increasingly high standard. The roads, what there are, are good and are being extended further and further so this will increase the tourist trade, although travel by air is far quicker but obviously more expensive.

My hope is that the tourist trade is controlled and the beauty of this country is not overrun by thousands of tourists to the detriment of the country's environment.

We entered Botswana from Zimbabwe and the first town we arrived in was Francistown. We then travelled westwards towards Nata and Maun and passed through Toteng and then we drove along the north-western border of the Okavango Delta system towards the Panhandle of the Okavango River itself. The roads were good but eventually petered out shortly after leaving Maun, leaving a dirt track for us to continue our travels upon. Modern hotels are starting to appear, e.g., Riley's Hotel at Maun, where every comfort is afforded to the visiting traveller. This modern hotel is well worth a visit and has added attractions of a bar and swimming pool. Botswana is a land of great beauty where the wild elephant can still be seen roaming in the bush. It's attractions are many and it rekindles a sense of adventure in the traveller who ventures there.

OKAVANGO DELTA

The Okavango, the third largest river in Southern Africa, flows for a thousand kilometres through the Kalahari Desert and spreads out in a mighty delta. It is lush with flood plains, waterways, palm-covered islands and radiant with lagoons where blue lilies rise above a floor of dark green pads.

Kingfishers dart through the reeds or perch on papyrus reeds, hippos snort in the lagoons and elephant come down to the water to bathe and drink. Fishermen pole their canoes through the narrow waterways. It is a place where time seems to stand still.

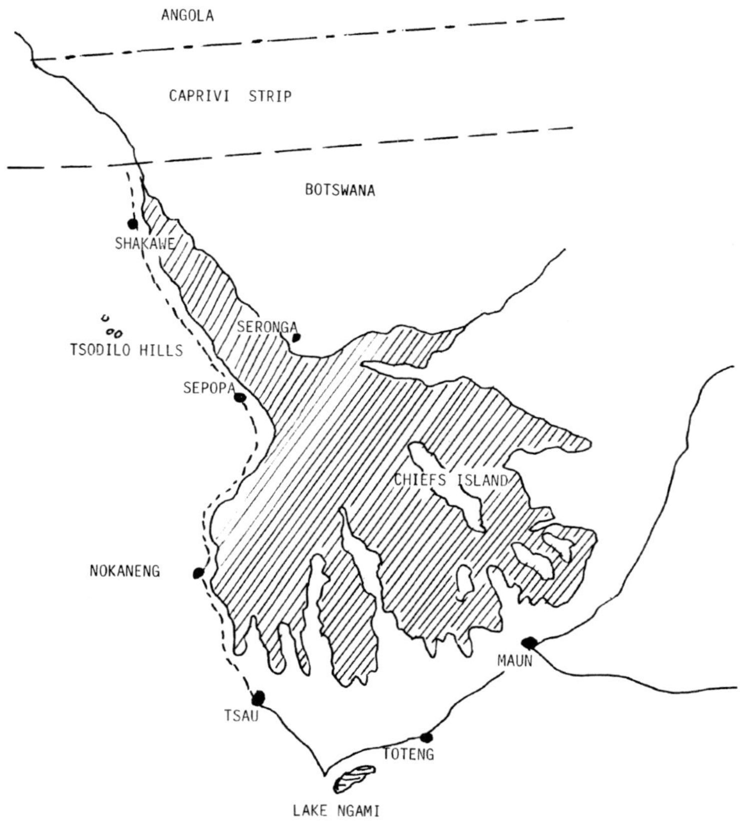

THE OKAVANGO RIVER AND DELTA SYSTEM

Each year as the rains end the Okavango rises and sweeps its way past Shakawe and spills over its banks. On its way it carries small islands of papyrus which have been broken away from river banks higher up stream. By June the flood is deep in the delta pushing through the reed beds and eventually flooding the open plains. As the water rises fish move into the shallows, ducks and geese arrive and crocodiles move into the water. By July the head of the flood has passed Maun and forces its way towards the open country to the southeast. The mighty flood is then gone, evaporated in the huge area of the Okavango Delta. What little water is left slips down into Lake Ngami.

Millions of years ago Africa slowly began to split apart. The crack or rift starts in the region of the Dead Sea and eventually disappears into the sands of Namibia. Today the edge of the rift is the east bank of the Malakane river in the delta system.

Water begins to flow into the delta in April just as the rains begin to finish. It brings with it millions of tons of sand and this is deposited to form a cone, with its apex in the north near Seronga. From Seronga the water spreads out and moves south-eastwards not necessarily in the main channels but extends across the flood plains and through the reed beds. The delta flood obviously depends on the earlier rains and the greater these are the more water eventually flows onto Lake Ngami. If the original rains are not great the flow of the river is variable. It is these changing flood patterns which give life to the delta and cause otherwise arid regions to be transformed into fertile land.

Much of the northern delta is permanently flooded and here grow vast papyrus reed beds which float above the sand and are kept open by the passage of hippopotamus, elephant and buffalo as they push their way from the main land to the islands and back again.

The lagoons are really oxbow lakes formed by the river bending back and forwards. Sometimes in the centre fig trees grow whose roots reach below the surface and whose branches bear the nests of herons and storks.

There are three major land masses which reach like fingers into the delta. The Matsebi in the west, Chiefs Island in the middle and Moremi in the east. This great variety of habitats, the Kalahari sands, permanent lagoons, forest and scrub, flood plain and reed bed make possible a wider diversity of animals than almost anywhere else on earth. Here hippopotamus, otter, and crocodile can live side by side with sable, zebra, giraffe and tsessege. Elephant and buffalo move freely from the drier habitat of the kudu and bat-eared fox to the wet reed beds of the lechwe and sitatunga. Constant changes in flooding provides feeding areas for the saddle-bill and marabou storks, pelicans, water-fowl and egrets. Truly the Delta is the home of wild life found nowhere else on earth.

Fishing was a popular pastime. Both tiger fish and bream were commonly caught. The former exciting to land and the latter delicious to eat. Fish were often brought into the camp site by the local children keen to sell them to us. As well as trying to sell us our next meal the locals were often spotted paddling their canoes up and down the river. Here they collected birds eggs, picked wild berries and of course fished. All their food was free all they had to do was to pick it or catch it - no such thing as the

ASDA shopping trolley for them! What a comparison there was between our respective life styles. We rush around from dawn to dusk trying to keep up with the clock, dash off to the shops after work and usually succeed in arriving home late! This was not the case here. Life passed slowly and quietly in a most spectacular environment. There were times when I felt most envious!

In the southern part of the delta system are three land masses which penetrate its lower region and here is found a vast array of different habitats. There are permanent sands, lagoons, forest and scrub, flood plains and reed beds and again a vast and extensive wild life is to be found. Here hippo, elephant, buffalo are all at home. Crocodiles and fish swim into the shallows and it is an environment where pelicans, water fowl, herons and egrets flourish.

The land here is rich and fertile and farming is very successful.

Medical problems among the members of the expedition kept me busy. Depression at home is bad enough but abroad can be heightened and poses difficult problems for the expedition doctor. There often appears no solution for the unfortunate patient in such a remote area and I spent many hours dealing with such a problem. In distant and far away places problems that have been submerged tend to surface with disastrous results and have to be dealt with in detail for the first time although they may have happened years ago. All this brought home to me how important it is for the expedition doctor to question closely eager young explorers before they leave home and then he may not be faced with difficult problems in the bush by a river in Northern Botswana. I suspect such problems are not common among the locals as they pursued their own particular gentle ways of life!

The Okavango river carries enough water to supply both England and Wales. It enters Botswana at Mohembo and then passes the village of Shakawe. From here to Seronga are the main breeding grounds for crocodiles which lay their eggs in holes scooped out of the sandbanks. As it enters Botswana the river is wide and broad and referred to as the pan-handle.

During low water from September to March the channel is fairly narrow but with the floods the reeds rise and the water spills over its banks flooding the surrounding plains. In the river are schools of hippos, otter, crocodiles and fish and in the reeds are sitatunga and a wide variety of bird life. Even I who am certainly not an ornithologist, counted forty different species of bird. The experts on the trip counted over a hundred and fifty. Along the banks of the river Hambukushu, Bayei and Batawana live by ploughing, keeping a few cattle, gathering wild food, hunting and fishing. Many of them still practise old crafts working with traditional tools, plaiting large mats, weaving baskets and working clay into pots.

On the banks of the river nest carmine bee-eaters in the their hundreds. While we were there we saw them tunnel their nests into the side of the river banks.

The earliest settlers of the Okavango Delta were the bushmen who have given their names to many of the islands and lagoons. About 500AD the first pastorolists began to arrive, settling in areas free of the tsetse fly. During more recent years people have come from all parts of the compass.

The first to arrive were the Bayei, poling their canoes through the shallows, tilling the flood plains and collecting wild plants to supplement their diet. Above all they fished with a variety of traps and nets. Overland from the south came the Bangologa desert dwellers who kept goat and sheep. These were followed by the powerful Batawana who eventually came to dominate the area. The Hambukushu came from the north moving south to avoid the slave traders. They became deep water fishermen, skilled with nets and spears. The last to come were the Hevero fleeing from the German war of extermination. In 1904 they rose against the German settlers in Namibia.

They inevitably lost their fight and fled into Botswana. They were initially subservient to the Batawana but eventually broke free of them and today are amongst the largest cattle owners. Their women still wear the long skirts and head-dresses introduced to them by the German settlers more than a hundred years ago. We witnessed this on a visit to Toteng as we left Maun on our way to Pan-handle of the Okavango near Shakawe.

Today much of the traditional way of life is still practised in the delta. Fish is the staple diet. As the water rises families set out into the heart of the swamp. Poling their canoes and taking with them their children chickens and belongings, they still till the soil of the flood plains and as the water recedes plant millet and cane. Wild food still forms an important part of their diet.

Maun is the capital of the Okavango and the gateway to the delta. A dusty sprawling village of about fifteen thousand people, it blends the new with the old. Modern offices and shops stand beside traditional homes of reed and thatch. An airport with a tarmac strip enables easy access to the delta region. There are schools, a modern hospital and the headquarters of the safari world. Maun is the road head but also the last step before plunging into the Africa of the 19th century. This state of affairs is not likely to remain for long. The road head will soon be developed to allow easier access to the Pan-handle region and tourism will expand into the more remote areas. I suppose this is inevitable but it left us with a feeling of sadness that so much of what we had been privileged to see would inevitably be changed by the march of progress. There are now fewer and fewer areas of the world that are being left undisturbed.

THE DOG THAT REFUSED TO DIE

We arrived soon after lunch one afternoon at the Shakawe Fishing Camp which is about five kilometres south of the village of Shakawe itself. The truck had become bogged down in the soft sand as we approached the camp having just left the main track. Here we were met by the owner of the camp in his Land-rover who had been informed of our plight. Eventually, and having wrecked the clutch we managed to free it and two hours later finally reached the camp site on the banks of the Okavango river. The camp site was started about twenty years ago by the present owners Barry and Elaine Pryce. Initially things must have been

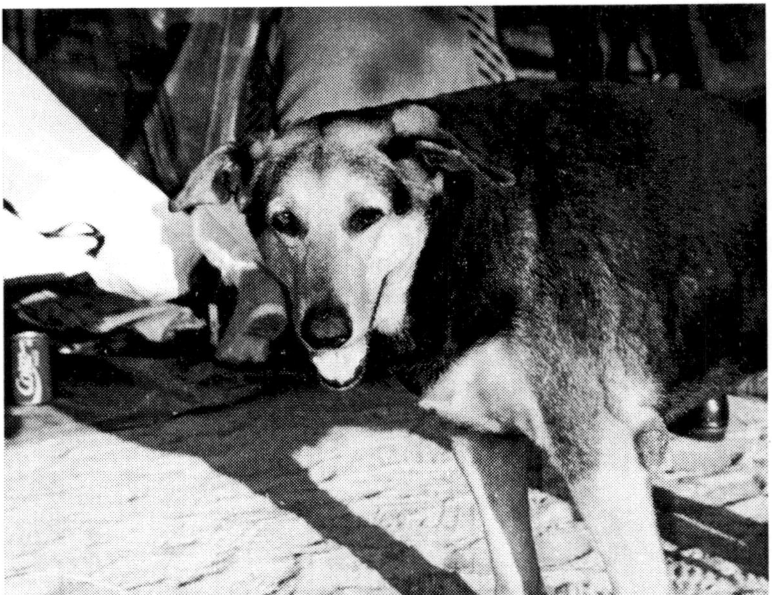

THE DOG WE TRIED TO KILL – 'LAZARUS'

fairly primitive but now, apart from camping areas, there are chalets to stay in, showers, a small swimming pool and a bar. The latter was the communal meeting place on the site and here I met Chris, an Australian doctor on the trip, in conversation with Barry and Elaine.

The Pryces had two dogs. A young Alsation called Tiger who was about four years old, an active and healthy dog. They also had a bitch called Tana who was elderly and presented a different sight. The bitch was as large as the Alsation but had some doberman in her as well. She was a pathetic sight, elderly and hardly able to walk due to advanced arthritis mainly in her hips. She whimpered when she walked, slowly and pathetically across the camp site and when she sat, or rather collapsed, it would take her an eternity to stand again. She had stopped eating and would only drink when encouraged. This was the topic of conversation as I entered the bar.

There was a pause at the end of the conversation and Barry Pryce looked up at us and asked if we would put his dog to sleep as he had seen it suffer for long enough. We looked at one another, looked at the dog and after further discussion reluctantly agreed to do it. 'I love dogs,' I said, 'we have always had one and ours has always been part of the family.' Putting a dog down is not an easy matter. 'Why don't you shoot the dog?' said Chris, 'we would certainly do that at home, it is quick and painless.' Barry looked up from the bar and replied that he had thought of doing it but could not bring himself to shoot his own dog. Chris and I went away back to the camp and worked out a plan to end the poor dog's days. We arranged to do it that night and told Barry Pryce of our intentions.

As we were talking late that afternoon around the camp, Tana slowly and painfully arrived and collapsed in a heap by the fire. We decided to do it there and then. We coaxed the dog slowly into the bush away from the camp site and when we had found a quiet place in the bush we lay the dog down. I can remember feeling sad and full of remorse, encouraging the poor dog to follow us knowing that we were going to try to end her days.

We found a quiet place in the bush, away from the camp site and lay the dog down on Chris's knee. I took my medical bag and a supply of brandy just in case. The brandy was for Chris and me and not for the dog. With the dog lying on Chris's knee we opened her mouth and gave an ample supply of sedatives and pain relieving drugs which we had mixed with jam that we had taken from the stores. We started this at about 6 o'clock and about three-quarters of an hour later the dog was sleeping and started to breathe irregularly. We then gave her even more sedation. About three-quarters of an hour later, the breathing became increasingly laboured and on several occasions she stopped breathing altogether but then restarted. We stayed with the dog the whole time, comforting it and stroking it. By this time over two hours had elapsed. Tiger the Alsation obviously realised that there was something amiss and had been there watching us from the start. He lay about thirty yards away. He came no closer to us and never left. I tried to encourage him to go but when he bared his teeth I decided that the dog was definitely staying. Now it was dark; behind us in the bush came a crashing noise; there were wild elephant near the camp site and I thought it had probably been an elephant. 'What the hell was that?' asked Chris, taking yet another gulp of the brandy. 'I haven't a clue,' I said and in the depressed mood that I was in I said that I really couldn't care less! Like a bolt of thunder and barking loudly Tiger shot up and came racing past us and vanished into the bush. There was a further commotion and eventually the Alsation appeared and silence reigned once again. The dog came over to where we were. We must have looked a pathetic sight, both of us feeling depressed and miserable. I have been in practice for more than twenty years but I have never felt as sad and miserable as I did that night. Tiger licked Tana's face and nudged her face with his and we couldn't believe our eyes. Tana's eyes opened and she lifted up her head! Chris and I were gob-smacked we couldn't believe it. There was another rush for the bottle of brandy. He is a tough guy, is Chris, at ease in the Australian bush and the previous year I had walked for two weeks with him across the Chalbi Desert, but his eyes filled with tears and I'm sure mine were also. This dog is not destined to die,' he said. So the four of us, the two dogs, Chris and I sat in a circle in the middle of the bush in the pitch black and reflected on the events of the past few hours.

Eventually, I said 'somebody will have to go and tell Barry that his dog is still alive.' I looked at Chris and the sadness and misery on his face had changed and he was showing signs of relief. 'I'm bloody glad the dog isn't dead,' he said. 'So am I,' I replied and once again we passed the bottle of brandy to each other.

I walked slowly back to the camp, leaving the three of them behind in the bush to find Barry Pryce behind the bar. 'Could I have a word with you,' I said, 'round the back.' In private behind the bar I related to him exactly what had happened, word for word, never lying or deviating from the truth and during this time held my head down. When I had finished I looked up and tears were rolling down his face. He put his hand on my shoulder, 'I'm so sorry,' he said, 'to have had to put you through that.' 'No problem,' I replied, 'I am just glad that the dog is OK.' 'So am I,' he said. 'Do you know,' he said, 'it's the most incredible dog I have ever known. I've pulled black mambas off the back of that dog. It used to protect people in the camp site and would even take them for walks in the bush.' There was a pause. 'I'll come round with the Land-rover,' he said 'and I'll bring the dog back here into the house.'

I walked back alone to the bush and we all then awaited his arrival. By this time Tana was still in remarkably good spirits. Her eyes were open but she still had her head resting on Chris's lap, being stroked all the time. We sat in silence and eventually finished off the brandy, relieved that the dog was still alive. 'Never again, Chris Jambor,' I said, 'never again will I try and end the days of a dog.' Chris looked up and with a smile on his face, 'I told you, you should have shot the bloody thing in the first place,' he laughed.

After about half an hour the lights of Barry Pryce's Land-rover came into view. He approached us through the bush and sat down. He must have sensed the atmosphere. 'I'm sorry,' he said once again. 'I'll take the dog back and meet you in the bar afterwards and we'll have a drink.' We helped him lift the dog on to a blanket in the back of his Land-rover. Tiger jumped into the passenger seat and the three of them drove off into the dark back to the camp site. Seeing that there was no more brandy to drink Chris and I trudged slowly back to the camp site and eventually reached the bar.

The story had obviously spread through the camp site and a few sarcastic comments were made, probably only in jest, but it didn't impress me and it certainly didn't impress Chris. Chris had a quiet word with one of the offenders and the so-called jocularity of the event was completely squashed. The bar had become quiet but slowly conversation was restored. The noise increased and the status quo in the bar returned to normal.

I saw Elaine Pryce come into the bar and I asked to have a word with her. I felt I owed her an explanation as well and once again described the events of the evening. When I had finished talking, it was obvious that the Pryces were equally concerned with our emotions as poor old Tana's. 'I am sorry,' she said, 'thank you for trying,' and then she paused, 'but will the dog be alright after all those drugs?' My simple answer was yes. Tana had had an enormous dose of drugs but in the back of my mind I had my doubts.

She smiled at me and I smiled back. 'Come on,' she said, I'll buy you both another brandy.'

We were still in the bar at 10.30 p.m., and had probably had enough alcohol for that night. Chris Jambor was smoking cigarettes by this time, something that he had never, ever done before. 'Come on,' I said to him, 'let's go and see Tana and make sure she's OK before we go to bed.' We walked out of the bar and down the side path to the Pryce's home. WE got to the door and struggled for ages, pushing and shoving. We then realised it was a sliding door and easily let ourselves in. We laughed and blamed the brandy. On a rug in the corner lay Tana, her eyes open, and as we approached her tail started to wag. We stroked and comforted the dog for several minutes and then aimed for the door and went back to the camp site. On the way back Chris Janbor said, 'you're a good bastard, Turner, you really care don't you; you'd make a fortune down in Australia doing medicine. 'You're not bad yourself,' I said 'for a bloody convict, but I'll tell you what, Chris Janbor, I hope you are better with your patients that you are with dogs.' We both laughed again and eventually climbed into our sleeping bags by the side of the Okavanga river. We listened for a while to the hippos snorting in the river and watched the stars shine in the African sky and then both of us drifted off to sleep. I remember thinking before I went to sleep that I was glad I was an expedition doctor and not a vet.

The next day, we both had a heavy head and whilst drinking coffee and eating breakfast Chris said to me, 'if we can't kill the dog, let's see if we can make its life a bit more bearable. We'll try some of the drugs that we use in the treatment of arthritis.' We sauntered off to the bar and told Barry Pryce what our latest plan was. 'Sure,' said Barry, 'I'll bring the dog over in the Land-rover and some her blankets so she can sleep by the fire.' We started the dog on drugs used in the treatment of arthritis, twice daily. We encouraged it to eat and drink and at night Tana slept by the fire. Slowly, over the next three to four days there was a remarkable improvement in the dog. She had lost some weight, she became more mobile and the pain was obviously less. Tana had regained some of her youth. We felt delighted; the Pryces were delighted and obviously the dog was too. Tana even started to go on short walks again, usually with Elaine Pryce as she went bird watching in the bush.

One night, whilst we were sat by the fire, the dog emerged from the dark of the night having been for a short walk.

Somebody gave her a biscuit and made her bed in front of the fire. After a pause somebody said, 'I see Lazarus is a lot better.' We all laughed. I remember thinking later that it wasn't just the dog that was feeling better, so did I.

We left the fishing village after another seven days and started the next part of our journey. This involved a three-hour drive along a dusty track into the Kalahari Desert to our next destination which was the Tsodilo Hills and here we set up camp once again.

THE GENERAL

The Tsodilo Hills lie in the northern part of the Kalahari Desert and are sacred to the bushmen. It is here that the bushmen believed that their gods live. There are four hills, a male, a female, an infant and a child, all close together. We were camping between the male and the female hill, adjacent to the bushmen's cave hidden in the female hill. About a mile further down into the desert the SAS were camping. I had met an army doctor from the SAS and his medical staff in the bushmen's village the day before and the other evidence of the SAS were their trail bikers who insisted on trying to drive through our camp one day.

It was about two o'clock in the afternoon and fortunately everybody was in camp. A convoy of armed vehicles started passing near the camp site and the Botswanian army arrived. Long-distance desert Land-rovers with machine guns at the front and rear and grenade launchers started to go past. Soon afterwards another party of troops arrived and started putting up camp about two hundred yards away from where we were. 'No panic,' said Peter. 'We will start worrying when the helicopters land,' and burst into laughter, when he saw the apprehension on our faces. True enough, about half an hour later helicopters started to land in the desert near the airstrip about two miles away. His expression changed for a moment. 'Stop worrying,' he said 'we'll really start worrying when the planes come in,' About three quarters of an hour later, planes started to land!

At first we thought there had been a coup or an invasion was about to take place as we were near the Namibian border. We tried to listen to the world service of the BBC but could gain no information. After some discussion we secured the camp as best we could and decided to go and try and have a look at the camp that had been set up by the Botswanian army. Fortunately, Peter agreed to do this. He returned in a bout ten minutes, short of breath. 'It's something serious,' he said, 'there's a Land-rover

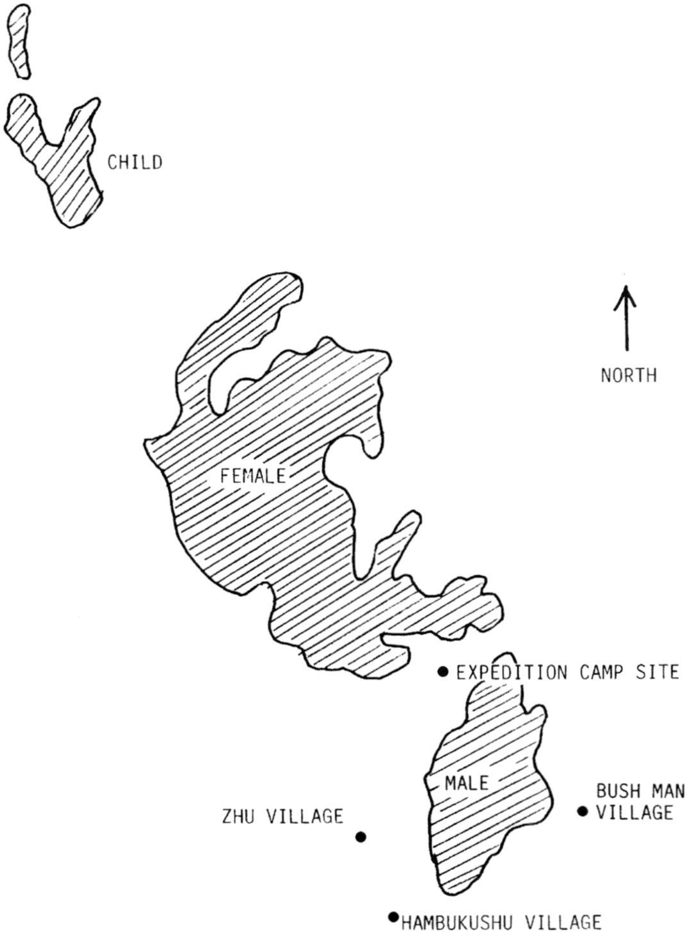

TSODILO HILLS

These are situated some 75km south west of Shakawe in the Kalahari Desert. The highest hill – The Male is – 1,300 ft and in this flat landscape is visible from a great distance. There is permanent water to be found and the bushman has lived here for about 20,000 years

over there with a fax machine in the back and they've just erected a satellite dish.'

Our next plan was to go to the SAS campo see if they could tell us what was going on, so three leaders set off into the bush to gather what information they could. We all waited apprehensively for their return and it wasn't long before they came back into the camp, in a state of some excitement. 'We are going to have a visit,' said Peter, from the English High Commissioner of Botswana and General Khama.' It turned out that the SAS and the Botswanian army were carrying out desert manoeuvres in a combined operation! Everybody was dutifully relieved and the odd nervous laugh and sigh of relief passed through the camp. We tidied the camp, organised the water supply and the kitchen and tried to make the camp look as neat and tidy as possible and efficiently run.

It wasn't long before two Land-rovers approached the camp site and the first two figures to enter the camp were the High Commissioner and General Khama. The latter was surrounded by four armed guards all with automatic rifles and not looking at all friendly. 'Look,' said on the members, 'they have small water bottles around their waists. 'Peter Drake smiled and in a quiet voice leant over to him and said, 'they are not water bottles you fool, those are grenades.'

Peter introduced the High Commissioner to all the members of the expedition and then started up conversation, talking about the Kalahari Desert and the Tsodilo Hills. 'Africa is my second home,' said Peter, during part of his conversation. There was a short sullen silence and General Karma, with his arms folded across his chest, looked him in the eyes and said, 'this is your better home,' in an intimidating voice. Peter readily agreed; in fact we all readily agreed with what the General had to say!

One of the purposes of the expedition was to locate the rock art which abounds in the Tsodilo Hills and draw up a plan of management for the area which we intended to present to the government of Botswana and this was discussed with our guests while they were there. After a short time they left to join the camp that they had set up nearby and we were all relieved by their departure as we had found the whole incident somewhat intimidating.

About an hour later, two soldiers appeared. 'The General would like to see some examples of rock art,' they said. 'Would you please come to our camp tomorrow morning at seven o'clock and arrange this for him.' This was apparently before the army manoeuvres departed the following day in the direction of the Okavanga river.

Jeff Carr and I were readily volunteered to go the next day to carry out the task. 'You must be joking,' said Jeff, but amidst the laughter of the others we were unanimously elected to go.

The next day we dutifully arrived on time outside the General's camp where the High Commissioner and the General were having breakfast. It was like being summoned to the headmaster's study and we stood meekly at the back of the camp with our arms clasped behind our backs. The General looked up. 'Come in chaps,' he said, 'take a seat. We are just finishing breakfast.' What a change there was from the day before. He was charming, courteous and obviously very interested in rock art. He grabbed a piece of toast and said, 'come on, how far is it to the nearest paintings?' 'There are two panels in easy walking distance,' I said. 'The first one is of rhinoceri and the other one is not far from it.' This was the panel of the dancing penises which I didn't mention to him at that time. I didn't push my luck.

The General and I strode out in front. He was definitely interested in what he was going to see. 'How old are they?' he asked, 'and who has done them?' I gave him what information I had learned about the rock art in the Tsodilo Hills and he seemed reasonably impressed. Behind followed his armed guards and Jeff and the High Commissioner until we eventually stood in front of the panel of rhinoceri. The General and his guards and the High Commissioner were satisfied with the information we had given them. 'There is another panel not far away,' I pointed out, walking over to Jeff Carr. I put my hand on his shoulder and whispered in his ear, 'I have shown him the rhinoceri, you can go and show him the panel of the dancing penises.' He smiled as he slowly crunched my foot under his boot. We eventually arrived back at the camp site about three quarters of an hour later. 'Would it be in order to take your photograph?' I asked the General. 'Certainly,' he said, 'would you like me to stand here in the sun?' 'Thank you,' said I and the photographs were duly taken.

As soon as they had arrived, they left and once again we were left alone in the Kalahari Desert. We stayed there for a total of twelve days - a management programme of the rock art was prepared. We explored and climbed the hills, visited the bushmen's village and finally left back towards the direction of Shakawe on the Okavango river before departing on the next part of our trip.

BUSHMEN OF THE KALAHARI

The bushmen of the Kalahari desert are the last survivors of a people who at one time lived all over southern Africa. They have lived there for over twenty thousand years. They first appeared in central and southern Africa and are a separate genetic race from the black Africans.

They pursued a nomadic way of life in virtual isolation. There was an abundance of game, water and rivers and a varied plant life for them to eat. Other areas were dry and cruel. They were fortunate that there was no other alien culture to disturb them and they existed with their own laws and ways of life. They had their own defined territories and spent most of their time hunting game and gathering food. Their survival, however, depended on their ability to find water. Bushmen are widely believed to be responsible for the rock art found in southern Africa.

The bushman is short in stature, about five foot in height with high cheekbones and a diamond-shaped face. He has an almost oriental look about him. He is lighter in colour than the black African and his body is lean and wiry. The hair on his head grows in tightly coiled spirals. The women are characterised by shelf-like buttocks and the males by semi-erect penises. These features are prominent in rock art.

About three thousand years ago another race similar to the bushman emerged. These were the Hottentots. They had the same ancestors as the bushman and had similar anatomical features. Their language was also similar. However, they added the herding of cattle to the hunter-gatherer way of life. They were also nomads but their movements were restricted by their cattle. They had a better diet and became more numerous than the bushman. They were better organised and elected chiefs and leaders.

Trouble soon developed as the cattle were responsible for dispersing the game upon which the bushman depended. The bushman started to raid the cattle, presumably initially to survive but later for convenience.

The bushman also came into conflict with the black Africans, the Bantu, and later with the Europeans who began to settle in southern Africa in about 1650. At this time the Portuguese started trading along the east coast of Africa and this created further problems for the bushman.

Later the British and the Dutch settlers arrived and trade started to flourish. This culminated in the formation of the Dutch East India Company and a further extension of trade.

The settlers brought with them cattle which brought them into further opposition with the poor bushman. Once again he raided and killed the cattle as he had done with the Hottentots, but real trouble erupted when he was held responsible for the

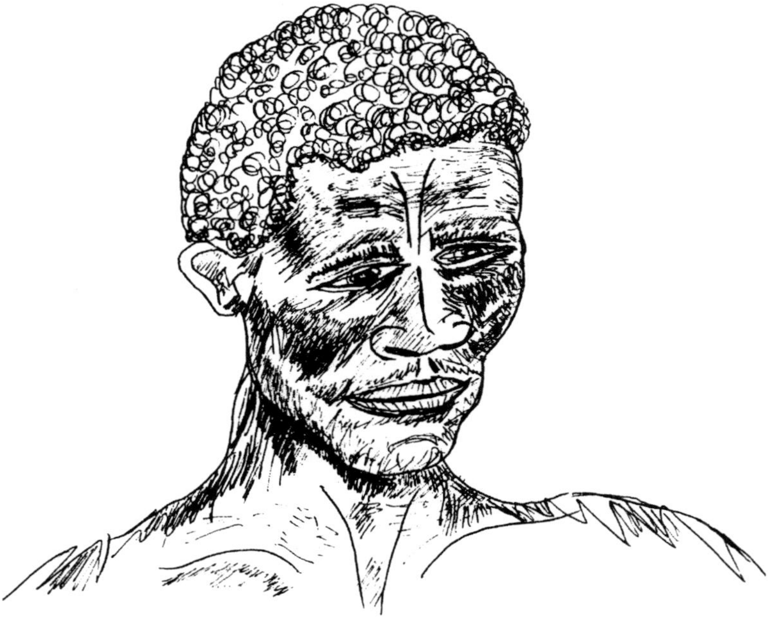

SAN OR BUSHMAN

The bushman was the original inhabitant in southern Africa and precedes the arrival of the black African. Few people can have been more misunderstood, and in the past was regarded as barely human and hunted and shot. He was however a master of survival in extremely harsh conditions having been forced to survive in the Kalahari Desert. He became a hunter, gatherer, his skills in hunting and botany were remarkable. His facial characteristics are unique and he looks as though he originated elsewhere. He successfully survived for thousands of years and was an expert in environmental control. For example, when collecting ostrich eggs he would shake them to ascertain if there was a developing chick inside. If there was he would leave it and only take what he needed. He is to be respected and admired for his achievements but fewer and fewer now live in the old traditional way. More of them are practising communal living, working on farms and near a stable water supply.

deaths of some Europeans on his raids. The Dutch farmers set up commando units with the specific intent of capturing and killing the bushman. Thousands were killed or captured. The captured bushmen were put in designated territories and they must have suffered a similar fate to the North American Indians in this respect. They were referred to as the tame bushmen as opposed to the wild bushmen who still remained free.

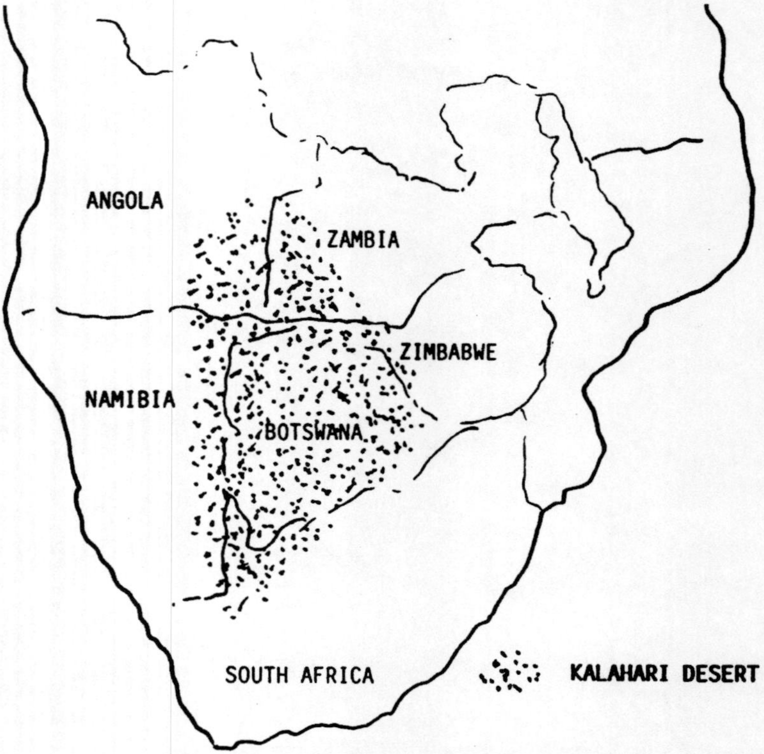

SOUTHERN AFRICA AND THE KALAHARI

The Bantu and the European settlers pushed further inland and further north and the bushman withdrew. They were eventually eliminated from southern Africa in about 1850. With all the odds stacked against him the bushman retreated to the only safe place he knew - the Kalahari Desert. This was an area so inhospitable that no one else could contemplate living there.

The Kalahari Desert is a vast basin of sand covered with bushman grass, scrub acacia and baobab trees. It extends some two hundred thousand square miles and most of it lies about three thousand feet above sea level. It did, however, provide for the bushman what he wanted. There was an abundance of wild game, plants and water storing tubers. There was wood for building huts, making fires, bows and arrows and also spears for hunting. There was, however, no running water at all - occasional standing water only. The average rainfall varies between eight and twenty inches and falls between January and March.

What does the future hold for the bushman? There are many questions to be addressed. How can he be helped to live in a modern day life totally alien to his former existence? What is in his best interests and should land be set aside for him? It should be up to him to decide his future but that depends on so many factors and I feel it will be difficult for him to maintain his dignity, independence and freedom in modern southern Africa.

Many of the bushmen now work for local farmers and have abandoned the hunter-gatherer way of life. Probably only about a thousand live in the traditional way out of a total of about fifty thousand.

The bushmen lived in huts and small communities but they did not live too close together. Their survival depended on water and they became expert in gathering and storing water. Water was usually collected in ostrich eggs. They used a sipping stick to collect water from trees where it had collected or from the ground. They also obtained water from plants at certain times of the year but this was the bottom line of survival. The bushman was an expert in travelling great distances. He carried ostrich eggs filled with water in a sack on his back. He left water dumps at certain points and then returned later the same way. This was a technique he used when raiding cattle. The bushmen never accumulated any property or wealth and were usually on the move looking for game or water.

He used fire-sticks for lighting fires. The base was of soft wood into which a notch was cut. Into this a hard piece of wood was rapidly rotated and this produced a fine hot black dust. This spilled onto dried grass placed underneath. The bushman would pick this up and gently blow until the grass burst into flames. A fire was kept most of the time especially at night. It was used for cooking and keeping warm but it was also a focal point where people could gather and discuss matters of common interest.

He seldom slept in his hut. It was mainly for storage and ostrich eggs filled with water could be kept cool here. They usually travelled around in groups of about twenty to forty and had owners who were in charge – these were representatives of the whole group. They had no defined chief or leader as did the Hottentots.

There was an equal balance of opinion between men and women and both shared the work depending on its nature. Men would undertake the heavy manual work. Arguments were settled amicably usually by separation and later by reconciliation.

Women gathered plant food – beans, berries and roots. They used a digging stick to collect the latter. The commonest root they used as a source of water was a form of wild turnip. It was shredded and squeezed and the water drunk as it trickled from their hands. The remainder of the root was used for washing their hands and faces. They also found a variety of onions, potatoes and truffles. In this way the women developed a high level of knowledge of botany and became experts at it.

Women seldom had more than two children. In a period of drought if a child was born it was suffocated. This is horrendous but it was a basic law of survival as regards the rest of the group were concerned. They breast-fed their children until they were about four or five years old. The care and bringing up of children was a top priority for the bushman and his family. When delivery was imminent the mother would go out alone into the bush. The baby was born with the mother in a squatting position. When the child cried the other members would go and look for her and bring them both back to the camp.

The menarche was of great ritual significance in the bushman community. At the start of menstruation the young girl was carried back to her hut where she was kept in the dark and wore neither clothes nor beads. No man was allowed to see her as this was regarded as bad luck. Outside men and women would dance and often go into a trance. When menstruation had finished the girl was washed and cleaned and then scarified across her shoulders and the middle of her chest above her breasts. Once this was finished she was dressed and led outside.

Before the white man came to southern Africa it must have been a natural paradise. There was a natural population control and the bushman would not upset or disturb the balance. When the white man arrived with his guns and ammunition there was a wanton slaughter of game. This had a disastrous effect on the bushman's way of life.

He had simple ways of trapping and killing game. He had developed the art of hunting with bows and arrows and used snares to trap his prey. The bow was made out of reed and twine. The arrow was in two parts – the head and the shaft. The shaft was made out of reed into which the head was inserted. The arrow heads were originally made out of bone but now metal is used. The twine behind the arrow head is impregnated with poison. This was obtained from the venom of puff adders, spiders and scorpions but the most lethal and effective poison was obtained from the lava of a beetle. These bows and arrows are still being used today as we discovered in the Tsodilo Hills. The bushman also used a throwing stick to stun small prey.

The eland was the most popular prey and they would go out hunting in groups of three or four. At a kill the successful hunter would eat the tongue but the rest of the meat would be taken back to the village to be shared amongst all the members.

It is a great shame this way of life is fast disappearing. Life today can be so much easier for the bushman and who can blame him for accepting it. However, he seems to have lost his dignity and I wondered if he was as happy as his noble ancestors had been. This was apparent to us when we visited the bushman village in the Tsodilo Hills. They had largely abandoned their hunter-gatherer way of life and survived largely by selling necklaces and bows and arrows to the people who visited them. Most of us had a feeling of sadness as we left the village.

ROCK ART

In the north-western part of Botswana near the border with Namibia lie the Tsodilo Hills. They are above a three hour drive from the Shakawe fishing village. There are four hills – the male, female, infant and child. The highest is the male hill some one thousand three hundred feet in height. These hills are holy to the bushman and it is here that they believe their gods live. They refer to them as the copper mountains which is a description of them as the sun sets over the Kalahari Desert and the hills glow red-orange in colour. It is in these hills that a wide range of rock art is found, predominantly on the female hill. It was the major project of the expedition I was on to locate and identify the rock art and present to the government of Botswana a management plan for the area. We discovered many forms of rock art, most executed with red dye and depicting animals that were familiar to the bushman. Eland, gemsbock, zebra, rhino, elephant and cattle. Most of the panels depicted animals but human forms were also evident. The latter emphasised the anatomical peculiarities of the bushman – the shelf-like buttocks of the female and the semi-erect penis of the male. It was in the Tsodilo Hills that we met Alec Campbell.

Alec Campbell is a well known authority on Botswana and a world leading authority on rock art. He had been excavating and digging in the Tsodilo Hills for many years and as we sat on the ground around his latest excavation site he gave us a brief insight into his knowledge of the area.

Rock art attributed to the bushman has been found all over southern Africa. The date of the earliest paintings is not known. In Namibia art has been found dated at 25,000 years of age. It was probably started in Africa about 60,000 years ago. It predates European art and is made up of different art creations.

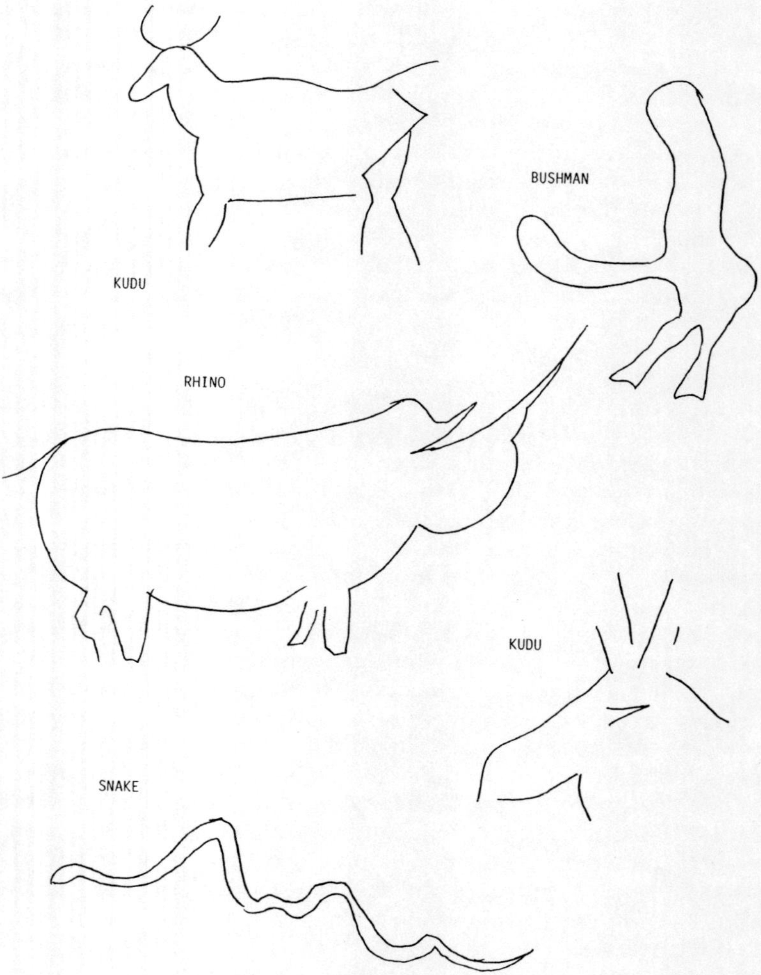

EXAMPLES OF ROCK ART

The first inhabitants to join the bushman in the Tsodilo Hills probably came from the Congo region – probably at the time of Christ. They brought with them goats and sheep, they made pottery and hunted and fished. They also traded in copper and iron and chains have been found containing these. Earrings have also been discovered and sieves for sieving salt.

In about 600-700 AD another group arrived from the Zambesi and settled in the hills. There is evidence of major trade interaction. Stone tools have been found, as well as ostrich egg necklaces and glass beads. All this is indicative of close-living communities.

Rock art predates the arrival of the black African and was carried out by the bushman. Many impressions of animals have been found – cattle, kudu, elephant and ostrich. Different forms of rock art have been found but paintings of cattle predominate throughout the spectrum of paintings and they must all have been done at a similar time. Paintings have also been found in East Africa and Zambia which are similar to those found in the Tsodilo Hills.

Some aspects of rock art are thought to have been influenced by religion. There are examples of schematic rock art experienced by the bushman whilst in a trance. The trance was initiated by dancing. It was during these trances that the bushman would try to communicate with his gods who he believed were capable of bringing rain.

Most of the rock art is characterised by red dyes. These were produced from iron oxides which are mixed with animal fats and blood. The people used sticks, feathers and their hands to paint the rock after first smoothing the area with a stone. When he had finished the bushman would often leave his hand prints as a form of signature.

Art produced using white dyes is also present in the hills but it is the black African who is responsible for these and not the bushman.

We discovered a wide range depicting both animal and human forms. We were, however, disturbed to find there was no plan to protect and preserve this unique area. We found evidence of camping in close vicinity to rock art panels and litter lying around. It was of great concern to us that the area could be vandalised. Until a management programme is drawn up this area is at risk. It is part of the heritage of Botswana and also its future and everything possible should be done to preserve the area.

Once it has been damaged it will be lost forever.

It was our earnest hope that our ideas and plans for its management would be adopted by the government of Botswana. We formulated a trail guide through the female hill which passed by some of the most impressive rock art panels. Hopefully they will adopt some of our recommendations and preserve this most beautiful and so far unspoiled area of their country.

BENJAMIN AND HIS CHEST

I was playing my version of French bowls outside the entrance of the bushman's cave in the Tsodilo Hills and at the time was winning. I heard Peter yelling my name and when I had wandered back to camp about 200 yards away I found him talking to an elderly bushman. 'This is Benjamin,' he said and he has been coughing for several weeks and losing weight. Benjamin had been deep in conversation with Peter and was telling him how the Tsodilo Hills came into being. There are four hills in the Tsodilo range in northern Botswana and this is the story he told. He pointed over to the male hill which is the largest and said that at one time it was a man. This hill was a man who had two wives and loved the second one more than the first and a quarrel broke out between the husband and the first wife. One day she took a stick and hit him on the head and he pointed towards the hill again. She threw down the youngest child and ran off on her own. After some time the Great God saw that the first wife was alone and went to the man and asked him where she was. The husband told him of the fight. The god was annoyed and said that because they could not live in peace, it would be better if they were turned to stone and so the man became the big hill, the first woman became the hill that stands on its own and the children became the hills in the middle. When he had finished his story he started coughing and spluttering and became very short of breath.

I asked him to take his jacket off which had been given to him by one of the members of the expedition.

I lifted up his shirt to listen to his chest. Benjamin had a right basal pneumonia and together with the long-term cough and his losing weight I suspected he had pulmonary tuberculosis, which is common in Botswana. I gave him some antibiotics but explained that he really should have his chest X-rayed to try and confirm the diagnosis. Peter agreed to take him the next day to Shakawe and there they could arrange for this to be done. He stayed and talked for a while and then left. We hoped to see him the next day but he never turned up.

What stories he could have told us about his life as a bushman all those years ago. His mind must have been filled with countless stories about his hunter-gatherer way of life in the Kalahari Desert. That elderly bushman must have been a mine of information and his survival skills must have been outstanding. I hoped that his basal pneumonia would respond to broad spectrum antibiotics I had given him and that it was not the tubercle bacillus that was the cause of his chest complaint.

RENAL COLIC AND THE CRACKLING GRASS

I had just returned from walking in the Tsodilo Hills where we were trying to make a trail in an attempt to preserve the rock art that abounds on the female hill. I was asked to come and look at one of the girls who was lying on her camp bed and obviously in a lot of pain. She was lying on her side doubled up in agony, clutching right loin. After a few questions and a quick look at her abdomen I realised she was suffering from renal colic and had a stone in her right kidney. On more direct questioning she revealed that she had had kidney problems as a child, I suppose with being dehydrated in the desert a kidney stone had formed and the result was there to see. I gave her some sedation to help her rest and ease her pain and enlisted one of the other girls to act as nurse for the day. There was no shortage of willing volunteers. I reviewed her later in the evening and all was well.

At about two o'clock in the morning my nurse for the day was shaking my shoulder. 'Come on,' she said 'she is in pain again and crying.' I tumbled out of my sleeping bag, grabbed my medical rucksack and found her in a similar state to the one in which I had found her before. By the light of a torch I gave her further sedation and stayed with her until she went to sleep.

About half an hour later the girl who had been her nurse the previous day said that she thought she could hear the grass crackling. We both listened carefully and sure enough the grass was crackling. We shone the torch and saw the surrounding grass area was alive and as it moved it was certainly crackling. I shone the torch closer to reveal millions of ants on the march. The rest of the camp was soon awake and we kicked and swept the grass away from the camping area. I have never seen anything like it in my life before; ants were everywhere. We soon brought everything under control again, cleared the remaining grass away, built up the fire and once more settled down to sleep. My patient had slept through the whole incident!

The next day she was fine and was instructed to drink as much fluid as possible. I advised her on her return to see her GP to have her kidneys X-rayed to make sure there were no more stones. I also wondered the next day what might have happened if I had not been disturbed that night. African ants in your sleeping bag cannot be much fun!

SHAKAWE MISSION HOSPITAL AND HIPPO ATTACKS

Whilst in Botswana I visited the mission hospital at Shakawe on the banks of the Okavango river. As you entered the village the hospital was on the right-hand side opposite the police station. It was stone built with a wooden roof and on benches outside the main entrance sat rows of the local people waiting to be treated by the nurses who worked there. It was here that I found myself late one morning. The girl with whom I had gone had decided to visit the local school while I decided to see the mission hospital. I knocked on the door and introduced myself to a young nurse who was running the clinic. She seemed apprehensive and uncertain at first but soon relaxed and started talking about the patients she had to deal with.

The hospital was run entirely by nurses and only visited once a month by a doctor. They were locally trained girls from Francistown. They worked as nurse practitioners and the work they carried out was of a high standard. They took histories from patients, made a diagnosis, carried out simple investigations and prescribed treatment. There was also a well stocked dispensary in the hospital where patients could pick up their prescriptions.

The main ward had two beds, both occupied when I was there. An elderly man had a chest infection, probably tuberculosis and in the other bed was a middle-aged lady with burns on her leg. There was a single-bedded labour ward where the nurse had delivered twins that same morning. There was also an adjoining lying-in ward. Obstetrics was obviously of major importance here. Along the corridor was a small kitchen where friends or relatives could cook meals for members of their family who were in-patients. Further down the corridor was a clinic room and a small area cordoned off for performing minor operations.

I sat with the nurse on duty and helped when asked to help her deal with problems that presented themselves. They were mainly kids with coughs and colds, similar to general practice in England. This I discovered was the commonest reason people attended the clinic which surprised me at first. Other problems more specific to Botswana were also evident and included malaria, sexually transmitted diseases, tuberculosis and malnutrition.

I was asking the nurse who accompanied me for the morning what casualties they had to deal with apart from the usual cuts and bruises. 'We do have a problem with hippo attacks,' she remarked out of the blue and my face must have shown some surprise as she then went on to tell me more. Hippos are wonderful to watch as they laze and grunt in the river and the noises they make at night are magical, but they kill more people in Africa than any other animal. They're big and cuddly but do not place yourself between water and a hippo as they cover short distances with amazing speed. So much for the stories in children's books where they are portrayed as loveable and cuddly animals. They can be lethal.

She told me what to do if I was the subject of a hippo attack in the water with a smile on her face. 'Dive under water downstream,' she went on, 'and at the same time remove an article of clothing. You then swim to the surface and throw this at the hippo, the idea being that it will play with this instead of you. You should then make your way to the river bank and return home.' I started laughing and replied that that was all very well 'but what if he does not want to play with your shirt and what about the crocodile on the banks looking for an early lunch?' She smiled back at me and we both ended up laughing together.

The fate of the hippo in the Okavango is in the balance as they are ruthlessly hunted and killed for food by the local tribes. Not as you may think with a bow and arrow from a canoe, but with high-powered rifles from craft with outboard motors. Conservationists in Kenya are worried about the fate of the elephant and rhino but in Botswana their concern lies with the hippo.

I was full of admiration for the nurses who worked in the mission hospital. They worked largely unsupervised, made important clinical decisions and the responsibility they undertook was high. They were cheerful and hard working and obviously proud of the work they undertook. I did not blame them – they were great. Whenever a patient came to the hospital they carried with them their own medical card. This was updated by the nurse on duty and a record of her diagnosis was entered. Children up to the age of five carried a pink card and adults had a blue one. The immunisation rate amongst the children was extremely high and they were encouraged to attend the clinic regularly.

I spent most of the morning and early afternoon in the clinic and the time flew by. I thanked the nurses for their kindness and they even offered me a job, but it was time for me to go, so having met up with the girl who visited the school, we both returned to the camp site at the Shakawe fishing village.

CHINA

The land mass of China is enormous and as a consequence there are extremes of climatic conditions. In the south the winters are warm but in the north the opposite is true and the conditions are bitterly cold in the extreme. China boasts the highest mountains; there are deserts, fertile plains, pine forests and tropical rain forests. All the world, it would appear, in one nation. In the north it is bordered by Mongolia and Russia, to the west by India and Pakistan and Nepal. In the west by Korea and the islands of Japan. Its eastern coastline is extensive and along the southeast aspect lies the island of Taiwan. Most of the population live in the eastern part of the country where the larger cities are found – Beijing, Nanking and Shanghai. In such a large land area and in such a diverse environment there are many different races and political views. The population of China is enormous and family planning is high on the list of priorities. One-child families are the norm and any breaching of these rules is liable to severe penalties. Certainly the young Chinese doctors we spoke to only had one child and were all too well aware of the risks of not conforming to this law.

China's written history dates back some four thousand years but the discovery of the Peking Man revealed that primitive man lived in China 400,000 years ago. It was largely left undisturbed for many centuries until in the sixteenth century the first Europeans arrived in the form of the Portuguese. After them came the Spanish, Dutch and the British and they inevitably brought with them trade, missionaries and, from a medical point of view, disease. The Chinese were not unnaturally suspicious of this threat to change and trading ships were subject to strict regulations. The Chinese refused to import foreign goods but were very happy to enjoy a thriving export market, especially in tea. The led to trouble, as you may expect. China had received financial gains in silver from its exports and to try and redress the balance the British imported opium as a way to balance the financial problems. This erupted into the first Opium War – 1839-1842 at the end of which China had to pay large sums of money in compensation and open up its ports to foreign trade. However, all was not well and the second Opium War raged from 1857-1860.

It seemed that at that time China was up for grabs and ran the risk of being split up into foreign hands in a similar way to the fate of Africa. Opposition groups emerged largely in the form of the Boxer Movement. However, this was defeated and brought to heel but it did succeed in bringing about a growing national pride and identity.

In 1928 Chiang Kai Shek took over as president of China and China took a much firmer hand in the control of its destiny. After the Second World War, having fought on the side of the Allies and against Japan, China was accepted as a power with equal rights. Things began to move in China with help from abroad, but between 1931 and 1935 Chiang Kai Shek had to face and sort out the merging threat of communism. This party was led by Mao Zedong and it was he who eventually rose to power in 1949. He proclaimed that the Chinese people had risen again and communism succeeded in uniting China. I have stood on the balcony of the gate for heavenly peace where those words were spoken, overlooking the vast expanse of Tianenman Square. All was relatively quiet on that cold November morning but the atmosphere must have been electric on that momentous day.

From that day China became united in a common aim and all

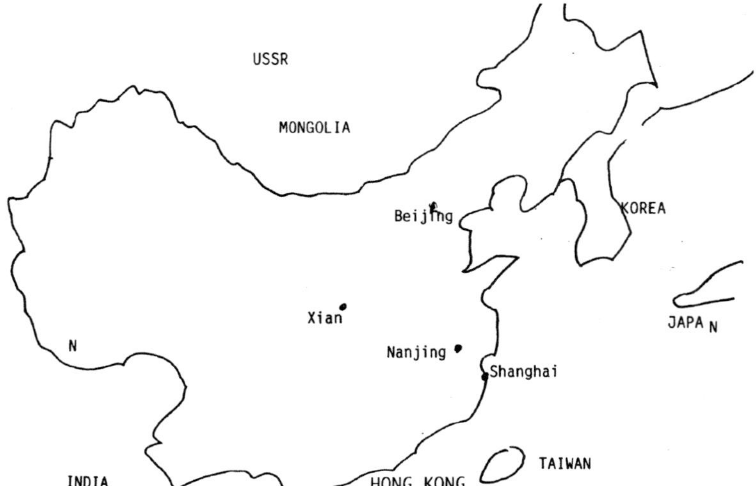

CHINA

people were equally involved. Civil war had left the economy in ruins; there was no modern industry and China was regarded as one of the world's poorest countries – but apparently all that was about to change. Millions of peasants were given land, huge amounts of money was poured into creating a modern industry and the Peoples Republic of China set up its grand Five-Year plan to change the face of China and bring prosperity to all. Unfortunately this great leap forward fell well short of its intended goal. Once again discontent emerged – the promises of a bright future collapsed. Mao Zedong tried to counteract this by setting up The Great Peoples Cultural Revolution with the emergence of the Red Guards whose purpose was to suppress opposition. This partially succeeded and communism prevailed. After the death of Mao and the collapse of the Great Leap Forward, Deng Xaioping came to power and communism fell rapidly into disrepute so a more democratic way of life emerged. Free trade was permitted and religious freedom was granted again. Today Li Peng is the prime minister and the problems he faces are enormous – the population explosion, student unrest, the demand for western goods and an even more democratic way of life more akin to western ideas. Change at the moment is rapid as we witnessed during our stay, but the secret of success must lie in the ability to control its rate of progress. The student revolts will certainly emerge again but unless China moves forward as one with each party recognising the other's problems, more storm clouds will gather and may break, with devastating results.

ACUPUNCTURE AND LIU WEI JUAN

I was feeling fed up one afternoon, at the time reading one of the medical journals, when my eyes landed on an opportunity to go to Beijing in northern China to study acupuncture at the Academy of Traditional Chinese Medicine. The address I had to contact was in Oxford so I didn't bother to write but rang them up instead. I spoke to a Chinese doctor, found out what was going on and four weeks later attended a symposium on Chinese Medicine at the University of Oxford. The subject of acupuncture fascinated me and I was anxious to learn more. On my return home I wandered off to the local library and book shop to satisfy my curiosity. Five weeks later in November I found myself sitting in the Academy of Traditional Chinese Medicine in Beijing.

'To understand Chinese medicine you should try to forget everything you have learned about western medicine and, unless you understand them both fully, never try to combine them.' Those were the opening remarks of Professor Cheung, head of the academy. The professor was of slight stature, dressed in a navy blue suit with a high collar with sandals on his feet. His hair was grey, as was his long thin beard and as he smiled at us he revealed his nicotine-stained teeth. He is a most eminent physician and a member of the World Health Council. He is a most dedicated and caring doctor completely committed to his profession and is surrounded by his team of enthusiastic young doctors, all equally committed.

Traditional Chinese Medicine goes back at least five thousand years to the Stone Age in China. Stones used in the early practice of medicine have been found – the Bian stones. They were used to incise abscesses and were also used in blood-letting according to some theories. The Bronze and Iron ages followed and needles made of iron and copper have been found in tombs believed to have been used in acupuncture, also bamboo and ivory needles have been discovered. Early drawings of meridian lines have been found printed on silks and tortoise shells. Acupuncture precedes Western Medicine by thousands of years.

At one time China was a collection of many races and customs but at about the time of Christ it was united by its first emperor and has become what we recognise as China today. Philosophers and teachers were prominent and the most well known were Confucius, Mung and Dao. It is in Daoism that the early theories and concepts of traditional Chinese medicine were first documented and organised. These involved the theories of Yin and Yang, the five elements, the concept of Qi – pronounced Chi a vital energy force which passed along meridian lines on the surface of the body, and the function of the Zang-Fu organs. Even at this time the Chinese understood the workings of the heart and other internal organs. This was even more remarkable when you realise that dissection of human bodies was forbidden by the Chinese as this would prevent the spirits of the body reaching heaven, or the more evil spirits to the Yellow River.

The Chinese believe that the internal organs are connected internally and externally by meridian lines and each organ has its own meridian line on the skin. These have to be learned. It is on these lines that exist some 365 acupoints named after rivers, architectural features, animals and some medical terms. By stimulating these points the flow of Qi is restored to the internal organ that is out of balance and once restored the organ can heal itself. It is based on a concept of balance and harmony within the human body and if this is upset illness follows. The aim of acupuncture is to restore this balance.

YIN-YANG AND THE FIVE ELEMENTS

These two theories were the two interpretations of all natural phenomena that originated in early China and not unnaturally the early Chinese Physicians adapted them to traditional Chinese Medicine. Yin and yang reflected all the forms and characteristics that existed in the universe and were the laws of heaven and earth. Put more simply they apply to two opposites of whatever you may decide to study for example day and night. Day is warm bright and is yang – on the other hand the night is dark and cold and is yin. The idea of Yin and yang is however not absolute but relative and one never totally dominates the other, they are dependent upon one another but are constantly changing. So at dawn they are in balance but as the day progresses yang becomes dominant and at mid-day is at its maximum and then starts to wane as afternoon and then dusk arrives. It is then that yin comes into dominance and reaches its maximum at mid-night and then the cycle is completed again at dawn. It is a question of balance being maintained even though great changes are going on. Providing the balance is maintained all is well but if the balance is upset then trouble follows.

The Five Elements refer to the five categories that exist in the natural world and were the most relative to the early Chinese.

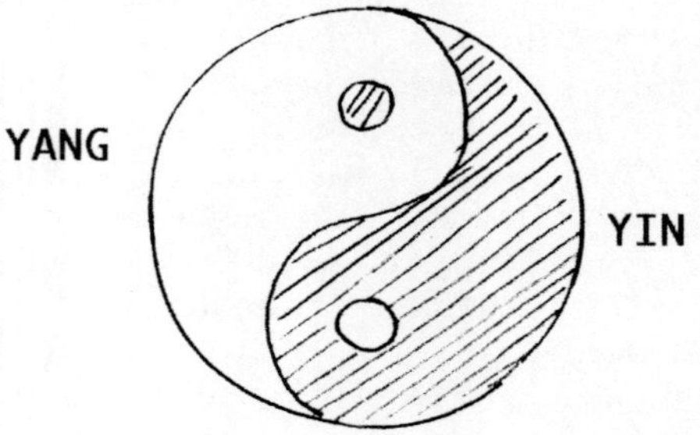

Although different they are all interconnected and depend upon one another. They are wood, fire, earth, metal and water. Wood is needed to make fire, the fire burns and what is left is returned to the earth. The earth gives up its metal and water and the latter is needed to make wood and the cycle is complete. These two theories were adapted by the Chinese Physicians to the twelve internal organs or as they described them the Zang-Fu organs. These were paired with the elements except that of fire to which four were credited.

The Chinese understand disease and illnesses as being caused by external factors, namely the wind, heat, cold and damp, but also internal factors including anxiety, worry, grief

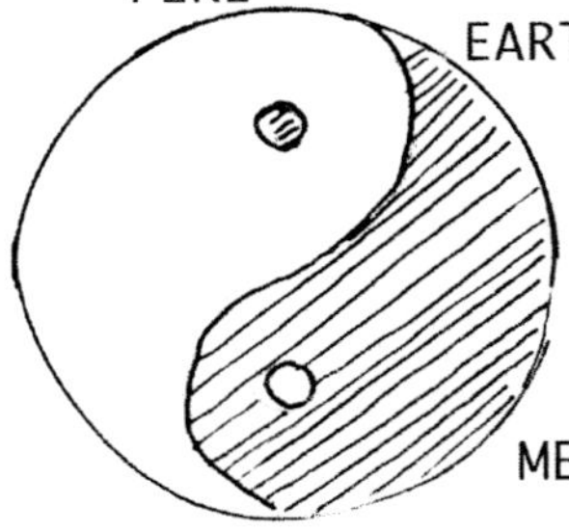

anger and jealousy. The latter certainly are pertinent to modern western ideas from some thousands of years later. The Chinese physician made his diagnosis by looking, smelling and above all, by careful examination of the pulse. Each of the internal organs is represented on the pulse and this brought Chinese Medicine into conflict with western ideas. The Chinese physician will examine the pulse from some minutes up to hours before reaching his diagnosis and once the cause of the illness has been discovered and which organ is involved, the treatment is directed to the meridian lines involved by needle acupuncture.

There is no doubt that western medicine has made astounding gains but it seemed to me that there were gaps that could be plugged by traditional Chinese theories. They have many appealing lines of treatment, they treat the body as a whole, drugs are not used; their medicine is relatively easy to understand and perform and there is little in the way of side effects. However, if I fell off a wall and broke my leg I would not be rushing off to a Chinese physician, but if I had intractable pain due to arthritis, migraine or had unexplained abdominal pain my outlook might well be different.

We stayed at a hotel in the northern part of Beijing in an older part of the capital. It was very comfortable, with all modern amenities. We were up at seven each morning and ate breakfast on the streets from street kitchens selling dumplings, pancakes soup and fruits. All very enjoyable and very cheap. The street cooks were very interested in our presence and one morning when we did not turn up they all expressed interest as to how we were and why we had not arrived that day. After breakfast it was back to the hotel, leaping on our bikes and cycling the short journey to the academy. Here we were met by a taxi and taken to the university hospital in the centre of Beijing. Here we attended out-patient clinics for two weeks learning the art and practice of acupuncture. Everything was treated by acupuncture; asthma, gall bladder disease, skin diseases, bed-wetting, malignant disease, migraine, headaches and a wide range of orthopaedic problems. Every patient had a history taken, a diagnosis made and the treatment consisted of needle acupuncture, ear acupuncture, moxa burning, massage and herbal remedies depending on the condition involved. By the end of our stay, with the help of an interpreter, we were doing the same. Embarrassingly wrong to start with, but at least with some success before we left!

On our first visits to the clinics, although we were treated with courtesy and respect, there was still a barrier between us and the Chinese. I recognised that unless we could break this down we would not learn as much as we might have, if things had been more relaxed and friendly. The next day we turned up with sweets, biscuits and flowers and having shared these and made the doctors laugh at our antics we continued on a much more friendly and relaxed basis. It certainly paid dividends and our relationship became much more agreeable.

It was here in the clinic that I met Liu Wei Juan. She was in her early thirties, dressed in her white clinic coat, but the most beautiful thing about her was her smile. When she smiled her face came to life and fortunately she spent most of her time smiling. She had been trained in both western and Chinese medicine and had spent several years studying paediatric cardiology before deciding to enter the world of traditional Chinese medicine. She was married with one son and proudly showed us her family photo album. She was always very keen to show us needle techniques and explained many of the mysteries of Chinese medicine. Under her guiding hand we progressed fairly rapidly and we learned much during our relatively short stay. Every day was a joy in the clinics and I was dreading the day when we would have to leave. Inevitably it arrived and once again we turned up with sweets and biscuits to celebrate our last day. The time soon arrived when we had to say our good-byes. 'You make us very happy,' Liu Wei Juan said. 'You are content.' 'I am also happy and content.' We are sorry to see you go.' It was an incredibly moving occasion as I shook hands with her and I could not resist giving her a hug before I left. All the other doctors lined up to say farewell and we shook hands with them all as they queued at the door to the entrance of the clinic room. Never would I forget my experiences in the University Hospital of Beijing.

During our stay we visited the Summer Palace, Tianeman Square, the Forbidden City, the Ming Tombs in the north and walked along the Great Wall of China. China is a fabulous place to visit and great changes are occurring rapidly. Student unrest is rife and at the moment rigidly suppressed. The shops are full of electrical goods. Volkswagen are building a car factory; young Chinese business men carry mobile phones. The worry must be that, although the cities will progress rapidly to a more western way of life, the vast majority of Chinese peasants will be left far behind. The streets heaved with people, most of them on bicycles, with traffic ploughing a furrow down the middle. Food is plentiful and we ate in local restaurants. I did not ask what was on the menu but remembered the words of my health visitor before I left, 'the Chinese eat everything with four legs except tables,' she had laughed. Snakes, frogs, sparrows, dog, puppy, chicken and fish were all on the menu. My stomach survived all onslaughts!

My memories of China are mainly reserved for the people I met during our stay. Whether you practise western or Chinese medicine you have one common aim and that is caring for people who are sick. The theories and methods are different but the aim is the same. There is no doubt in my mind that both forms of medicine have much to learn from each other. We should listen more to each other and respect our different views and then perhaps we will each gain from sharing different experiences and knowledge.

THE LITTLE GIRL WHO WET THE BED

Each day started at about seven a.m., a quick shower and onto the streets for breakfast. Fruit, pancakes, dumplings, soup and sweet potatoes. The sweet potatoes were the most popular. The streets in Beijing are alive at this time in the morning and the food kitchens do a roaring trade feeding the locals and the occasional visitor. After satisfying our appetites we trudged back to the hotel, leapt on our bikes and headed in the direction of the Academy of Traditional Chinese Medicine. It was a short journey of about ten minutes but not without its hazards. Having left our bikes locked up outside the lecture building we wandered to the front entrance to await the arrival of the taxi which then took us to the University Hospital of Beijing where we attended an out-patients department.

Beijing appeared to be a sea of people – some twelve million people live here. The pavements and roads heave with pedestrians, bicycles and traffic. Bicycles pass four lanes across on either side of the road and traffic ploughs a furrow down the middle. Policemen on duty try to do their best to control the chaos. Fortune favours the brave in the Beijing traffic. The fatalities for cyclists are horrendous. As you can imagine, travel is very slow and not without its risks! The journey to the hospital takes about thirty minutes.

The entrance to the hospital was characterised by a mass of people streaming into the hospital entrance. Patients were brought by their relatives on carts and stretchers often towed by bicycles. There is no ambulance service as far as these people are concerned! We were soon swept into the hospital and jostled and fought our way to the out-patients clinic. It was here that we presented ourselves each morning during our stay.

The patients presented themselves with a wide range of problems – asthma, high blood pressure, gall stones, duodenal ulcers and aches and pains of every sort. The patient who stole my heart was a little girl of about six years whose problem was wetting her bed at night. She was immaculately dressed in trousers and a blouse and a brightly coloured jacket but she was obviously frightened though she managed to keep her composure. After taking the history and examining her the treatment prescribed was a combination of needle and ear acupuncture.

Her concerned mother led her child to a cubicle and laid her on a couch to await the arrival of the doctor. Acupuncture needles were inserted into her abdomen and leg and during this time a loving mother held her child's head in her arms. The needles were left for about twenty minutes and then seeds were stuck onto her ear which was the prescribed treatment with ear acupuncture. All this having been done the child and mother presented themselves for the final assessment.

As she stood before us I could not resist reaching into my pocket for some sweets that I had brought for such an occasion which I gave to her along with my biro. I spoke to our interpreter and asked him to tell her that the sweets were for being brave and the biro to help her with her studies at school. The message was duly passed on and for the first time she smiled and spoke to me in Chinese. The other doctors roared with laughter and the mother looked somewhat embarrassed. Our interpreter put his hand on my shoulder and smiling said the little girl had said

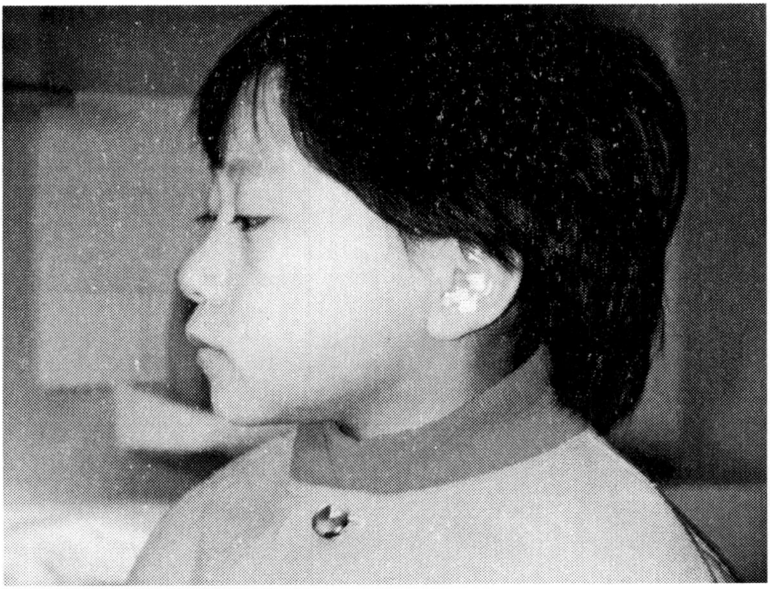

THE LITTLE GIRL WHO WET THE BED
The plasters on her ears are examples of ear acupuncture

'Thank you, grandfather!' We all laughed together eventually, including her mum.

As the laughter died down the mother bent down and whispered in her daughter's ear. The child smiled and then her face became serious and she took a pace back and went through the routine of physical education Chinese children are taught at school. One foot forward and then back and to the side with her arms raised to the side, then over her head. The whole performance was beautifully executed and took about two minutes. We all clapped in approval. The little girl was obviously well pleased with her work and I gave her some more sweets. She soon disappeared out of the clinic into the crowd of patients outside and we carried on with our mornings work. By the end of our stay we were taking histories, making diagnosis and treating patients.

It had happened to me again! I remembered Ali Ben Braheim in the High Atlas and the young Samburu boy in Kenya. All these moments had been magical and all we had done was to care for each other. We came from different parts of the world; we spoke different languages and had never met before but those precious memories will always live with me. Anyway, what had she meant – bloody grandfather indeed!

THE FOURTH MUSKETEER

I thought hospitals in England were busy but these are nothing compared to the site I witnessed in Beijing. The place heaved with people; patients sat on wooden benches outside clinic rooms, those who could not sit stood or leant against the wall. Doors opened and closed and white-coated doctors scurried around.

At first many Chinese came to our clinic more out of interest, having heard about the foreign doctors than anything else but towards the end of the first week few patients came as by this time we were treating patients by acupuncture ourselves. The message had obviously spread!

It was during one of these periods of quiet that Dr Liu suggested we should go and watch an elderly Chinese professor practise his own style of acupuncture. One that he had perfected over many years, but she warned us that it was different to the way we had been taught and different to the accepted, more modern method.

We were led along the corridor, tiptoeing between the waiting patients, and found ourselves in a small clinic room. It was here we were introduced to the elderly physician. The professor must have been in his late sixties, small of stature, grey haired and slightly bent which gave him a stooping posture. He was dressed in a white clinic coat, was clean-shaven and had sandals on his feet. He smiled at us and made us feel welcome. He was obviously very popular as there were many patients waiting to see him. Once again our interpreter explained that this was a different type of acupuncture but this warning in no way prepared me for what was about to happen.

We had been taught that acupuncture needling should be done carefully, gently and precisely. Once the needle had been inserted under the skin the needle – about two inches long – was slowly raised up and down until the patient felt a feeling of warmth or an ache. When this was obtained it was an indication that the flow of Qi had been found. The Chinese referred to this procedure as 'Fishing for Qi' – the vital energy force that flows in the body. Once this had been ascertained the needle was either rotated in a clockwise direction to re-enforce the flow of Qi or rotated in an anticlockwise direction to suppress the flow. If the flow was excessive the needle could also be swayed to allow the energy force to escape. This was referred to as 'Swaying the green dragon's tail.' In some cases a herb – Moxa – was placed on the needles and burnt. This was used to treat illnesses caused by the cold and the damp. It was commonly used in treating arthritic conditions. All these manoeuvres were worked out in advance and performed slowly and with considerable care. It was also impressed on us that it was important how the needle was removed. Slowly if Qi was excessive and quickly if the flow of Qi was deficient. What we were about to witness paid little homage to these methods.

The patients were questioned as before and then laid on the examination couch. Instead of lying flat they were positioned on their side in a curled-up position. To my utter amazement the elderly physician approached the patient with a needle some six to eight inches long and, having ascertained the correct site, plunged it deeply into the unsuspecting patient. The needle was left only for about a minute, not the twenty minutes we had usually witnessed and then it was suddenly withdrawn. I felt sick as he repeated the procedure several times.

I could not believe what I was seeing. My mind automatically thought of the complications of such an action. We nicknamed him the fourth musketeer! The patients seemed to feel little pain as the needle passed deeply inside their body – I cringed! The whole procedure was done with great speed and much activity.

Our interpreter must have seen the look on my face, and put his hand on my shoulder and started laughing at me. 'Cheer up' he said. 'He has been perfecting this method of acupuncture for over fifty years,' and he pointed out there were many patients waiting to see him. I then calmed down a little.

As I recovered from this experience I studied this remarkable man even more closely and realised he was an expert in his field – probably the only one! The doctor must have seen the look of astonishment on my face and I felt somewhat embarrassed – and much to my apprehension he took my arm and brought me to the side of the patient. She was a young Chinese girl of about twenty years of age. He spoke gently to the young girl and then to my horror placed his long needle in my hand and pointed to the place on the skin into which I should insert it. I looked across to our interpreter who had his hand across his face and obviously found the whole situation highly amusing. It's OK for you, I remember thinking. There was little else I could do. With great speed I tried to copy the method I had been introduced to ; stuck the needle deeply into her side, twisted the needle – left it for about twenty seconds and then with great gusto pulled it out.

The professor seemed reasonable pleased with my efforts but I was only too glad it was all over! We stayed for about another fifteen minutes but it was with great relief that we returned to our own clinic room. By this time it had filled up again with patients during our absence!

The whole incident caused me much concern and occupied my mind for the rest of the day. At least I had done it! If I were to practise this type of medicine at home I would be locked up and certified as probably insane, not fit to practice medicine and struck off the medical list, but here was an eminently experienced and respected doctor who was popular with his patients and held in the greatest esteem. It's a crazy world sometimes!

ACUPUNCTURE ANAESTHESIA

We visited general hospital wards during our stay and witnessed the treatment of stroke victims. Physiotherapy certainly played a large part, as did herbal medicine and needle acupuncture. We were escorted around a cancer hospital by a young Chinese surgeon and were shown the different methods of treatment that were available. Western medicine has certainly had an impact in China and most patients had been subjected to surgery, chemo and radio therapy. Chinese medicine was much in evidence especially in relation to the treatment of the side effects of such treatment. Herbal medicine played a large part in this regard. The most memorably trip, however, was to a neurosurgical unit on the outskirts of Beijing where we witnessed the benefits of acupuncture anaesthesia.

This is reserved for adults over the age of sixteen, it is more commonly requested by the more elderly and peasant communities and nobody with a history of fits is taken on. All patients have the opportunity of a general anaesthetic if they wish and this may be granted once the operation has started. It is largely reserved for Caesarean Sections, thyroid surgery and neurosurgery.

The benefits are obvious; the patient is conscious throughout, there is no risk of dealing with an unconscious patient and the recovery rate is rapid, with little in the way of post-operative complications. The doubt that must remain is whether the level of pain relief is acceptable?

Once clad in operating gowns, masks and sandals on our feet, we stood in line in the neuro-surgical theatre where an elderly man was having a pituitary tumour removed. There were three acupuncture needles in his face and two in his right foot. His pulse and blood pressure were monitored throughout, as was his heart rhythm. He had been given drugs to help him relax and to relieve his pain but throughout the whole procedure he was conscious.

The surgeons injected sterile water under his scalp and then lifted the scalp from the skull. Having done this they drilled four holes in his skull and lifted this up revealing his brain underneath. The senior surgeon then entered the theatre, took control and successfully removed the brain tumour.

I was absolutely flabbergasted and could not believe what my eyes told me I was seeing. At one point the patient raised his hand and I rapidly dispatched our interpreter to find out what was the matter! It turned out that the patient said he was feeling a little sick. So much for the patient – what about the western doctors who were watching! After the operation he was helped off the operating table and taken back to his hospital bed.

There is no doubt acupuncture anaesthesia works; I saw it with my own eyes and nobody in their right mind would subject himself to such pain if modern anaesthesia were available. I imagined that the patient might start fitting or lose consciousness, but no such problem emerged.

How sensible it seems to me to take the best of both western and Chinese medicine and use them for the benefit of the patient.

THE CALL DURING THE NIGHT

Being on call during the night is not one of the more appealing aspects in the life of a busy General Practitioner. Having worked hard all day and with the prospect of another one to come an undisturbed nights sleep is welcome indeed. It is the telephone that summons me to the patients bedside – a mum worried about her child or a patient with pain that has not settled. Armed with the name and address of my patient, my medical bag and having reluctantly crawled out of bed I venture forth into the night. Snuggled up in my jacket and scarf I switch the car heater up to make my journey more comfortable.

It is not always easy to find the correct address. Numbers on house doors are frequently missing. There is no light to guide you and certainly nobody on the street to greet you on your arrival. Having knocked on the door there is often a lapse in time before the door is eventually opened. Having gained entry and having spoken to the anxious relative I climb up the steep stair case to the shown the patient. A few minutes later having ascertained what the problem is and the diagnosis made, the treatment is left to tide the patient through the night and a suitable follow up arranged. The days are long gone when the doctor was shown to the bathroom to wash his hands after examining his patient or escorted to the front door and thanked for his attention.

If everything in my mind is settled and I am happy with the diagnosis I repack my medical bag, head for the front door, stepping over the dog and hopefully will soon be back at home in a warm bed. It is my earnest wish before dropping off to sleep that I will not be woken until the alarm clock goes off in the morning. I occasionally reach the stage after a busy night when the alarm clock bursts into activity that I pick up the telephone and announce 'Hello – this is the doctor, can I help you?' I am sure even that reaction would have confused Pavlov and perhaps I have been doing night work for too long!

Life was not so for the early Chinese Physician. It would not be the telephone that would arouse him from his slumbers more likely urgent knocking at this door. Struggling through the dark with the aid of a candle and opening his door he would have been confronted by the disturber of his sleep. The man would bow and beg his forgiveness for disturbing him at such an hour. The messenger would likely be the servant of a wealthy land owner whose wife had been taken ill suddenly in the night. Having invited him in the doctor hurriedly dressed, collected his acupuncture needles, herbal medicines and also a small doll to help him in making a diagnosis. He was then escorted to a waiting carriage to take him to his patients side.

His journey would certainly have taken him longer but the owner of the house would be waiting to greet him outside and the house ablaze with light in the darkness of the night.

He would be escorted to the patients bed side, a chair placed for him to sit on and then he would be left in private. Questions would be asked pertinent to Chinese medicine but during this time he would not be allowed to see his patient being separated from her by a heavy curtain. When he had finished his questioning he would then pass his hand through the curtains and feel her pulse for many minutes to help him make his final diagnosis. He would also pass the doll to the patient and ask her to mark in crayon on the doll where she felt the pain. When in possession of all this information he asked the patient to place her arm or leg outside the curtain and insert his needles at various acupoints to restore the balance of Qi to enable his patient to recover. This whole procedure may have taken over an hour to perform. Having finished and collected his belongings, refused a cup of tea he was then escorted to the waiting carriage to be taken home and finally his bed.

As he approached his house lanterns would be burning outside, each one representing the death of one of his patients. Obviously the fewer the better, but the less there were the more likely he would be called out at night! All Chinese Physicians had to obey this decree of the Emperor and the penalties for not doing so were severe.

So having related these two stories I pondered to myself as to who had the better deal. Both of us had been awoken from our sleep and my journey would have been quicker but I suspect he spent more time out of bed than I did. However I would submit that my days were far more busy than his. He was certainly treated with more respect than I and was taken to and from his patients home and met in the street on his arrival. The advantages of Western Medicine are obvious to me and I do not have to carry a small doll to help me make a diagnosis and I am able to see my patient. I certainly do not have to hang lanterns outside my surgery to inform people how many of my patients have died! The comparisons continued to intrigue me and I found great difficulty arriving at a decision. At the end of a practice meeting one evening I related my problem to my medical colleagues. The general consensus after a great deal of discussion was that both came out of our experiences about equal. It would appear that some aspects of medicine change very little despite the passage of time!

A COMFORTABLE WAY TO TRAVEL HOME

I was reluctant to leave China and return home. In the past when home is in sight I heave a sigh of relief, but this time it was different. Although I love the excitement of travel it gives me great satisfaction to return home to family and friends and I suppose I am fortunate in this respect, but this time my experiences had been unforgettable; it had been akin to watching television for fifteen days, interesting, stimulating and a completely different experience which I had adapted to very quickly. I had seen a completely new way of life, different attitudes and priorities and also experienced a completely different diet. I had set off from home with some feelings of hesitation but they were soon dispelled.

The flight left at seven o'clock in the evening and we arrived at the airport in plenty of time by courtesy of a car from the Academy. We were left at the departure area and made our way through the usual procedures. The departure area was modern. Indeed, in fact, so modern that parts of it were still being given the finishing touches. We paid our airport tax, booked our seats and had our baggage weighed. We soon found ourselves in a large customs-free shopping area, but to my dismay it was closed so we trudged along corridors to the departure lounge and awaited our call to board the plane to take us on our long eighteen hour journey home.

On board I found to my joy we had been given seats in a exit area and I could stretch my legs on the way home. I had an interesting book which I was reading and settled down to a relatively enjoyable trip. Travel by Air China was comfortable indeed – drinks, a meal and then settled down to watch a film courtesy of the Chinese travel agencies. I then began to get lost in my book.

We had been travelling for about two hours when I saw a man trip up in the aisle on his way to the toilet area. My first impression was that he had probably had too much to drink and once again delved into my book. About ten minutes later I realised he was still there, although he was mainly hidden from view and felt I should go and find out what was going on. I excused myself to the two travellers who were between myself and the aisle and saw the man still collapsed surrounded by anxious Chinese air hostesses. They obviously had not a clue what was going on. As I knelt down beside him I realised the seriousness of the situation. He was unconscious, no pulse, shocked but still breathing. My first thoughts were that he had had a heart attack and was dying and urgently summoned his travelling companion. Nothing happened. I once again enquired about his family and soon an anxious lady appeared from the back of the aircraft. I asked her many relevant questions and concluded he had had a form of fit or faint. As it turned out, he had suffered similar attacks before. By this time he was fortunately regaining consciousness and once again I asked him a barrage of questions which confirmed my original diagnosis. By this time a young girl was kneeling by my side who turned out to be a nurse who worked in an intensive care unit in England. I related to her what had happened and what conclusions I had come to . This seemed an ideal situation to improve my flight home even more.

After a pause I whispered to her to agree with everything I said and to do as I suggested. I turned around to the line of apprehensive air hostesses and enquired if any of them spoke English – one of them assured me that she did. 'I am an English doctor,' I went on 'and know what the problem is here, but you must do exactly as I say.' This she readily agreed to do. 'We must move him to the first-class compartment,' I insisted, 'as he needs careful nursing and I will accept full responsibility for him.' Soon we were lifting him through to the luxury of the first-class area but once there she insisted that he sat on a seat presumably thinking about the comfort of the more expensive paying passengers. Once again I laid down the law and stated that unless she did as I suggested the responsibility would lie with Air China and not with me. We soon had made up a bed for him at the front of the cabin in front of two very comfortable reclining seats.

By this time the man was fully conscious and I found out more details about his plight. He had been suffering from gastroenteritis for two days and had lost a considerable amount of weight. He was dehydrated and obviously a very sick man. We nursed him and encouraged him to drink plenty of fluid. He hailed from Scotland and there ran a home for disturbed teenagers with the help of his wife. Eventually my friendly nurse and I sat in our respective seats and admired our new surroundings. It was great! On the opposite side of the cabin sat an Arab armed with a briefcase and behind us sat an English businessman on his way home from China. However, in the middle of the aisle stood a table, with an impressive array of alcoholic beverages and fruit juices. 'You must be thirsty,' I said to her, 'hang on, I will soon return.' I was soon seated next to her accompanied by a large fizzy orange juice for her and a beer and large expensive French brandy for myself. She rapidly downed three of these large orange juices and complemented me on my choice. 'Good,' she stated, 'really good.' 'So it should be,' I laughed, 'at home we call these Bucks Fizz!' Soon we both dissolved in laughter.

We cared for the man during our long journey home, often adopting a rota system, one vigilant while the other slept. We encouraged him to drink which he did, we ate first-class cuisine and enjoyed two video films. During the long flight the wife made several trips to visit her husband and was very grateful for the help we had given her husband. She obviously loved him very much. As we approached home again I asked one of the air hostesses to organise an ambulance to meet us at Gatwick Airport. This she did. Eventually we arrived at Gatwick. The plane was soon boarded by an efficient team of paramedics. I gave them a letter for the admitting doctor and soon the sick man was dispatched into an ambulance, heading for hospital with its lights flashing.

The travel couriers had been somewhat slow in their interest and I suggested to one of them that I would be sending a large bill for my services but decided not to bother as I was only too glad to have our patient home safe and sound.

The plane landed at seven o'clock local time and after passing through customs I soon found myself back at the long stay car park. After paying the bill I was soon heading north. The closer I drew to home the more excited I became and after about four hours I stood in the hall at home. Oh boy, I was home again. I sank into an easy chair and enjoyed the feeling of being home once again. I looked out of the window and saw Pendle Hill and the river Ribble below and China seemed a long long way away. No puppy or snake on the menu tonight, I remember thinking. I did not sit for long and was off again to retrieve the cat from the cattery and pick up the dog who had been staying with good old Wendy. A couple of hours later all three of us were seated in front of a log fire sharing fish and chips. Oh boy, it was really good to be back home.

SNAKES –

THEY STILL GIVE ME THE CREEPS

Whenever I saw snakes on the television I would dive behind the nearest cushion and wait until they had left the screen. When I visited Chester Zoo I cringed as I passed the snakes in the reptile house. I remember at school being chased by a boy holding a harmless grass snake. I would have won several events at the Olympic Games with the speed and agility I showed on that occasion. Realising that I would be coming into contact with snakes on my travels I endeavoured to find out more about them.

Everything I read seemed to confirm my worst fears. They were apparently lethal, definitely out to get you and once you were bitten you had had it and that was that! As I read further I developed a more reasonable attitude. They are not all bad news. They are responsible for restricting the spread of disease by killing vermin; they are a source of anti-coagulants used in medicine and when seen in their habitat look magnificent and command a great deal of respect. I discovered that they are not naturally aggressive; they were shy creatures and avoid human contact if possible. They are definitely not as they are portrayed in James Bond films.

In some ways snakes are the most interesting members of the animal kingdom. Without fins, they can swim with remarkable speed. Without legs, they can travel as fast as a man over short distances. Without feet some snakes can climb trees as rapidly as a monkey. Without hands they can bury themselves in earth or sand in a remarkably quick time. They can sleep without eyelids to close over their eyes, detect sound without complete ears, and eat meals that are larger than they are. Although they live close to the ground they are amongst the cleanest of animals. Despite all this they are probably the most misunderstood creatures in the world. So I was beginning to learn they were not as bad as I had once thought!

There are many reasons why it is difficult to get to know snakes. First, the pattern of their skin is excellent camouflage. You can walk past a snake without seeing it. They do not call out or cry and move slowly through the grass or bushes so they pass without being recognised. The shape of the snake enables it to crawl into hiding places without detection. Even in areas where snakes are common often the only thing that makes you aware of their presence is their discarded skin.

The idea that all snakes are dangerous is not true. By far the majority of the two thousand snakes in the world are harmless as far as humans are concerned, and only a few of the poisonous snakes will attack unless provoked or startled.

Snakes belong to a sub-order of reptiles called Serpentes. The temperature of their bodies does not stay at a uniform warmth and varies according to the temperature of the place where the snake stays for any length of time. This is the reason they are referred to as cold-blooded.

At first glance snakes seem to function like any other animal but there are specially adapted differences. The tongue of a snake helps it to smell and as it flickers in and out it collects molecules which enable a snake to follow prey for example. Their hearing is poor and they are far more likely to respond to vibrations on the ground than noise. So it is no use singing and shouting your way along in the bush as the snake will not hear you, but if you stamp your feet on the ground it will be aware of your presence.

So, armed with all this information, I ventured forth, but it was not to be all plain sailing. Although they will not attack unless provoked, some snakes are lazy and lie basking in the sun and are not very impressed when you stand on them. The puff adder is an example of this and is responsible for fifty per cent of the deaths from snake bites in Africa. So it pays to wear boots and watch where you put your feet. In dealing with snakes avoid them - it is quite simple, do not do as on a recent trip in Zimbabwe when two members of the expedition were poking a viper with a stick. Fortunately the snake had more sense than they did and shot off into the undergrowth. The rule in expedition medicine is simple. If you want trouble and go looking for it you will probably find it. Do not swim in rivers with matted vegetation around it. Do not go poking under stones, be careful where you decide to sit down and do not go poking your hand into undergrowth when looking for wood.

The first snakes I came across were in the Huri Hills. The person in front of me accidentally stood very close to two cobras who were wrestling with one another. This I discovered later was the way they fought and not as someone suggested, sexual attraction! They reared up and we both shot off in the other direction at a rate of knots. That was breaking rule number one - if you see a snake in close proximity stay still as the snake will strike at movement. I defy any life-loving person to stand still under these circumstances. So my first encounter ended in terror, fright and completely misjudging the situation. Full stop I vowed to do better the next time.

My next encounter with snakes was in Kalacha, the Gabbra settlement in northern Kenya. We had spent two days crossing the Chalbi Desert and could not believe it when we found there were showers there. They obviously proved very popular. Four members of the expedition had finished their shower but when the fifth went in he saw coiled up in a corner a deadly carpet viper. The snake was soon dispatched, not, I hasten to add, by me. I must confess it was the first time I felt sorry for a snake. It had crawled in to escape the heat of the midday sun, minded its own business and some kind soul had smashed its head in with a piece of wood. So much for snakes being aggressive.

When looking for a place to camp in the bush it was always Peter who would go in first to make sure all was safe. He used a panga knife to clear the area of unsuspecting beasts. We, as true and genuine cowards, would only venture in when the all-clear was given. You have to be decisive with snakes, he would say and any hesitancy was fraught with danger.

On my next encounter I made an even bigger fool of myself. We were sitting in the bar at the camp site on the banks of the Okavango river and spending a pleasant evening talking and drinking cool beer. I saw Peter peering into the corner of the bar under a low-lying table. He casually remarked that he could see a snake. I remember thinking it was probably the drink that had affected him but sure enough, out it crawled, heading in our direction. In true and gallant fashion I leapt onto the bar much to the amazement of the barman, who happened to be the owner of the camp site. Fortunately, one of the local farmers crushed the snake's head under his boot and threw it onto the fire. When I once again resumed my seat the look Peter gave me did not take a lot of working out to decipher! Failed again, I thought.

We then entered into conversation with the owner of the camp site. He told us he killed between ten and twenty black mambas every year on the camp site. My mind turned back to poor old James Bond, fast asleep with a deadly snake heading towards him, only to be brought back to earth by being offered another beer. 'I think it is time we went onto brandy,' I said casually and reached into my pocket for my wallet. Black Mambas are amongst the most dangerous snakes in Africa and there I was on an expedition apparently in mortal danger! I must be mad, I thought, I could be on a beach in Greece or Spain and here I am in snake-infested Africa. I followed very slowly and carefully behind Peter on our way back to the camping area, had a quick look in my sleeping bag to make sure nothing was lurking there and after a great deal of effort managed to drop off to sleep.

SNAKE BITES

You are strongly advised to admire snakes from a safe distance as they will not attack unless provoked. Snakes will strike at movement and if you see one it is advisable to stay still and allow them to slither away. It is important that members of an expedition use their common sense and do not leave sleeping bags and boots on the ground into which snakes may crawl. Snakes like to avoid the heat of the day and are often found in shower units or toilets so vigilance in these circumstances is to be recommended. When walking in the bush wear suitable footwear and walk slowly with a heavy foot so as to disturb snakes and enable them to escape. You should not in any circumstances corner a snake or it may attack and if a snake is killed do not handle it, as decapitated reactions can occur up to two hours later and you may be bitten.

The first snakes to evolve on the planet were the elapids and the modern day equivalent are the cobras, kraits and mambas. These fed on smaller reptiles and amphibians and the prey was killed by a neurotoxin and was kept in the snakes mouth and then swallowed. As evolution progressed the mammals appeared and these provided a different problem. They were larger and faster and it was then that the vipers appeared. They killed their prey by a haemotoxin. The snake could not catch the mammal but followed it until it died and then ate it.

The incidence of snake bites should be brought into a correct perspective. In some countries you are more likely to be killed by a coconut falling on your head rather than a snake bite! A poison from a neurotoxic snake attacks the nervous system with drooping of the eye lids, difficulty in swallowing, palsy, and there is little in the way of pain. The bite of a viper is more painful and affects the vascular system with spontaneous bleeding and bruising throughout the body.

I suppose if someone was bitten on the finger it may be theoretical to cut it off as soon as possible but this is impractical and not be recommended. Reassurance is most important and serious poisoning is rare and death highly exceptional especially if medical help is to hand. More harm is done to the patient by untrained staff than was ever done by a snake bite. Carefully

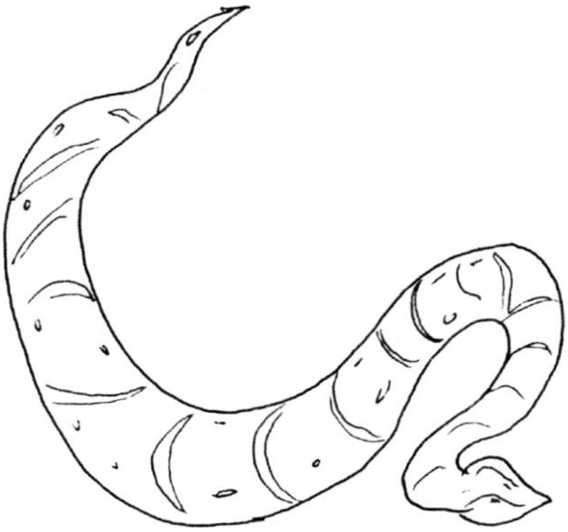

PUFF ADDER – BITIS ARIETANS 3' – 4'

This snake is found in Africa and is highly venomous. It is fat and sluggish and one of the longest vipers. It is a lazy snake and enjoys snoozing in the sun and will not usually slither off when you approach. Because of this you may well tread on it and run the risk of being bitten. It is the cause of the majority of deaths from snake bites in Africa.

wipe the site of the bite but some authorities would dispute this as they stress it may prevent identification of the poison. Certainly do not incise the bite as this only introduces infection and does not allow the poison to escape. Tourniquets may be used to prevent spread of the poison but should only be done if a large amount of venom has been injected. If hospital facilities are within half an hours journey then leave well alone. It is a good idea to apply a tight bandage over the bite and up the whole limb during transfer to a hospital.

If venom from a spitting cobra enters the eye wash it out as far as you can and urine may be one alternative to think about. If it is safe to kill the snake do so but do not run the risk of further trouble. The victim should be calmed down and then rested so as not to encourage rapid spread of the venom and then transferred to hospital as soon as possible. Preferably on a stretcher.

The use of anti venom on expeditions is not to be encouraged as its administration is not without risk and severe anaphylactic reactions can occur. Anti venom should only be given in hospital by experienced medical personnel and in an intravenous infusion.

If there is no swelling after a couple of hours the poor victim can be reassured but it is advisable to keep an eye on them for a further 12 hours. If it is a viper bite look out for abnormal bleeding and if an elapid bite look for signs affecting the nervous system. These clinical signs should be actively looked for and only when they appear should antivenom be given.

In northern Kenya I have heard local farmers describe how when bitten by a snake they passed an electric current through the site of the bite and above it. This was usually done with the help of a car battery or cattle prodder. This is not without its own risk and there is little evidence to suggest it is effective. It is more important to observe a common sense approach with reassurance, sedation and keeping the patient still.

All snake bites must be regarded as poisonous until proved otherwise. As stated most snakes are shy and will not attack unless provoked but the exception is the black mamba which is a territorial snake. Most bites are on the lower limb or hand but the mamba has a habit of rearing up and biting the trunk and is a most dangerous snake.

The mortality rate from snake bites differs regarding the toxin injected. In elapid snakes if sufficient venom has been injected it is about ten per cent and the average time of death varies from five to twenty hours. The mortality from viper bites is between one and fifteen per cent and death time up to forty eight hours.

As you can see I have done my best to find out more about this problem. Prevention is the key to success and discipline among the members of an expedition is important. I suppose most people have phobias about something but mine is definitely snakes. I suppose I could go on holiday to Greece or Spain in the future but somehow I doubt it. I would rather take my risks in beautiful and remote areas despite the problems I may encounter.

WHAT TO DO IF?

SOMEONE HAS GASTROENTERITIS

WE THINK SOMEONE HAS CONTRACTED MALARIA

SOMEONE HAS BROKEN A BONE

SOMEONE HAS A PANIC ATTACK

SOMEONE IS SUFFERING FROM HEAT STROKE

SOMEONE HAS BEEN BADLY BURNED

SOMEONE IS SUFFERING FROM HYPOTHERMIA

WE THINK SOMEONE MAY HAVE DROWNED

WE THINK A WOUND MAY NEED A SUTURE

SOMEONE HAS BEEN BITTEN

SOMEONE HAS BEEN BADLY INJURED

SOMEONE IS SUFFERING FROM SNOW BLINDNESS

SOMEONE IS SUFFERING FROM ACUTE MOUNTAIN SICKNESS

YOU ARE LOST IN A DESERT

SOMEBODY HAS BEEN EATING MY PORRIDGE

There are various medical conditions which may arise which should be discussed in more detail and information should be given as to how to cope with them. Gastroenteritis must be the top of the list. In all these conditions I cannot emphasise strongly enough that most of them are preventable and everything possible is done to minimise the risks. Members of an expedition should be aware of the problems that exist and have some insight into how to cope with them. Gastroenteritis is common; it may cause little in the way of problems but it can also proceed like wild fire with serious risks to health.

Gastroenteritis is characterised by vomiting, abdominal pain and diarrhoea and is an infection of the gastrointestinal tract. It may be caused by a variety of organisms bacterial, viral and parasitic. All produce the same picture but with some variations. For example, Campylobacter infections are characterised by severe abdominal pain and amoebic dysentery by bloody mucus stools. On an expedition it is not possible to identify the causative organism. This can only be done in the laboratory. It may appear that without knowing the cause of the illness you cannot do much to help but this is not the case here.

Vomiting and diarrhoea in hot climates can lead to rapid dehydration and treatment in this aspect has to be started as soon as symptoms appear, so action must be decisive. Fluid replacement is helped by the addition of electrolyte salts and must be given in small volumes often, rather than in larger volumes as these tend to be vomited back. Drugs to help to stop vomiting are useful and given by injection or now by buccal administration. Tablets to help to stop diarrhoea have limited value and your time is better directed to replacing fluid loss.

In hot climates gastroenteritis is often accompanied by a high fever and this rapidly accelerates the course of dehydration and again action in this aspect has to be early and decisive. Remove most of the clothing from the patient, lie them in the shade and liberally wet their body with water. Do not wipe it off but allow it to evaporate as this is how cooling occurs. This may have to be repeated on several occasions. Having brought the temperature down and started a management programme in respect of fluid replacement, it is important to isolate the patient and not allow him to return to his group as this will only encourage the spread of the infection. Doctors may be important on expeditions but not as important as nurses. Here the expedition nurse really comes into her own. If there is not a qualified nurse

I have found there are many willing volunteers to help in these circumstances.

Hopefully by pursuing your plan the outbreak will be brought under control. In my experience they tend to be rapid in onset, produce severe clinical disturbances but fortunately soon resolve. Antibiotics if there is a doctor present, are a useful tool to possess. Septrin-ciprofloxin and erythromycin all have their place, depending on the clinical presentation. Every doctor on an expedition should carry with him intravenous fluids as there may be an occasion when they may be used. If all else fails then admission to hospital may be necessary. This may all sound a little dramatic as the vast majority of sufferers make a complete recovery. The outbreak seldom lasts more than a few days and fewer than one per cent will develop prolonged symptoms. Most expedition members who have suffered gastroenteritis will have settle by the time they reach home. If however symptoms persist, the unfortunate patient should seek medical help and an attempt to identify the causative organism should be made. Then specific treatment can be started.

As I have stated before and, at the risk of appearing boring, prevention is far better than cure. There is no excuse for not maintaining camp discipline in the preparation of food, the serving of food and the disposal of food products. Gastroenteritis is the most common problem you are likely to come across and is almost inevitable, but if you act quickly and decisively the outbreak should not pose too serious a threat.

What do we do if we think we have contracted malaria?

Malaria is one of the most important tropical diseases with over 150 million cases and about one million deaths annually worldwide. Four species of malarial parasite have human hosts and are all transmitted by the Anopheles mosquito. The most serious is the falciparum form and may be fatal and is often referred to as malignant malaria. Most cases obviously occur where the mosquito is endemic but cases are often seen in non-endemic areas – the so called imported malaria. Certainly in Britain the cases have risen over fifty per cent in the last decade and as international travel increases this figure will presumably continue to rise. Not only may the traveller bring back malaria with him but the mosquito may have gained access to the aeroplane and may proceed to bite local residents, especially in the summer months. This is the so-called runway malaria.

The incubation period ranges from ten to forty days and depends on the species of mosquito. Other than a fever the symptoms are varied and none are diagnostic. The bouts of fever comprise three stages. The cold stage, followed by the hot and then finally the sweating stage. Having seen the clinical presentation it is only possible to diagnose with certainty by further laboratory tests.

So what do we do if we think someone has malaria? Remember that the incubation period varies from ten to forty days. Watch for the bouts of fever as described and if you think they fit the bill assume the patient has malaria and start treatment. It is far better to use your common sense and judgement and to do something rather than nothing. Giving someone anti malarial treatment certainly is not going to make them worse. The standard, very effective treatment is with oral chloroquine diphosphate. The adult dose is 600mg followed in six hours by 300mg and then 300mg on each of the following three days. Toxic effects from this drug are rare. In areas where resistance to chloroquine is prevalent quinine 600mg should be given in a dose of 600mg three times daily for seven days, plus fansidar three tablets at any one time during the seven days. The picture is also complicated by the fact that chloroquine resistance is only relative and in many regions where resistance to chloroquine is reported., chloroquine in full doses continues to be used successfully for primary treatment.

The risk of acquiring malaria can be reduced by a combination of three measures. Preventing the mosquito's access to the skin, deterring the mosquito from biting you and chemoprophylaxis against the malarial parasite. Stay indoors with screens on the windows, wear long sleeves, long trousers and socks and the use of mosquito nets at nights is easy and of proven benefit. Various insect repellents are available and these can be used on the skin, impregnated on clothes and mosquito nets. Chemoprophylaxis depends upon the part of the world you are going to and a regime should be instigated by the expedition doctor. The expedition member must be aware that no regime is fully protective and malaria may occur despite strict compliance. Whatever regime is used it must be continued for at least four weeks after returning from an endemic area and if symptoms arise that may suggest malaria urgent medical help must be sought.

There has always been much confusion in the treatment of malaria and regimes for treatment have often been changed. The hope in total and effective prevention lies with the development of a malarial vaccine and this is now under development, but its use will not be apparent for several years to come. Life will certainly be much more simple when this has been fully developed.

Within the past eighteen months the prophylactic treatment of malaria has changed again as regards travellers to Eastern Africa. Mefloquine or Lariam is now the drug of choice. The incidence of neuro-phschiatric side effects is in the order of 1:10,000. It is now recommended for areas of cholroquine resistance. Treatment for breakthrough malaria is now Halfan or Halofantrine given in three doses at six hourly intervals. I am not sure where this story will end as there are now areas in Africa and East Thailand where resistance to Mefloquine has been reported! It would seem that more attention should be directed to denying the mosquito access to the skin and ensuring that compliance with therapy is carried out correctly.

What do we do if we think someone has broken a bone or has a serious head injury?

The most likely injury is to the lower leg and ankle injuries are common especially on mountaineering expeditions. Again, wearing the correct footwear and using your common sense go a long way to preventing these. If a member is unfortunate to seriously injure his ankle and a fracture is suspected he has first of all to be examined. Carefully take his boot off if this is possible – if too much pain is experienced leave it on and assume it is broken. Strap it up; give him something to relieve his pain, for example, codeine tablets, and arrange for his evacuation and transport to hospital where the limb can be X-rayed. In examining the leg in a case of suspected fracture you are looking for extreme tenderness over the bone. The fracture may be obvious with deformity and the limb in a position that can only be seen in a fracture. On your first examination you may not be sure the leg is broken, therefore another look in a couple of hours is advisable. If in any doubt treat it as a fracture and act accordingly. Pain may be relieved by giving pain-relieving drugs but also by immobilising the limb in a splint.

Head injuries pose a different problem and must be treated with the utmost caution and respect. Any member who is unfortunate to suffer a significant head injury, for example, if he has been unconscious or the scalp is lacerated, must be assumed to have fractured his skull until proved otherwise and this can only be excluded by an X-ray. This obviously means transport to the nearest hospital. During this time his condition must be carefully observed to ascertain if his condition worsens. Most head injuries fortunately resolve with few complications however, vomiting is a symptom of severe injury as is the onset of drowsiness and more serious neurological symptoms, for example, epileptic fits all point to a serious situation. Every head injury must be carefully monitored and you are strongly advised to act on the side of caution. The fact that you may be made to look foolish and in fact the injury is not serious, is completely irrelevant. Someone has to make a decision and accept the responsibility. The best definition of responsibility I have come across is to make a decision with the information that you have available in the current emotional climate, knowing that you may be wrong! It is all well and good to make decisions with hindsight – that is easy. It is not so easy at the time. It is important to sit down, weigh up the facts, discuss them with your expedition leader and make a decision based on common sense, the vibes that you get, and not to act in panic.

Having related the seriousness that head injuries may present, the facts are that the vast majority of cases make a full recovery. You have to act sensibly because it is also the duty of the expedition doctor or leader to give an account of the injury to the parents or relatives of the unfortunate victim and you must be seen to have acted with care and decisions made in a sensible and realistic way.

What do we do if someone has a panic attack?

This is very likely to happen and common usually at the start of an expedition. People are tired, perhaps have not been to remote areas before and are disorientated in time and space. The most common presentation of a panic attack is hyperventilation. The patient is under extreme stress, whatever the cause and first of all experiences difficulty in breathing. Respiration proceeds faster and faster and the patient panics even more and this does not help his breathing problem. During this time he expires more and more carbon dioxide and this upsets the chemistry of the body and leads to tetany of the fingers and pins and needles in the body. By this time the unfortunate patient is in an even worse condition and convinced he is dying. It is the duty of the expedition doctor to look out for the likely candidates for this and be in a position to act quickly. All can be brought under control with a sympathetic approach and getting the patient to breathe into a paper bag held over the patient's mouth. This enables him to re-breathe the carbon dioxide, the chemistry of the body is returned to normal, the tetany or spasm of the fingers subsides and once again the situation is brought under control. Here again the expedition nurse comes into her own as the patient will need watching and reassuring over the next few days.

What do we do if someone suffers from heat stroke?

In the armed services sunburn is regarded as a self-inflicted injury and there is no excuse for any expedition member to suffer from the effects of sunburn. However, it is surprising how often I find myself reminding members of an expedition to cover themselves up and protect themselves from the sun. Discipline in dress is mandatory in preventing this. However, on every expedition there is usually one person who pays little heed to advice!

First of all, remove the sufferer into the shade and then start to tackle the main problems, namely burns to the skin, dehydration and the severe constitutional effects excessive exposure to the sun can produce. The body temperature can be reduced by tepid sponging. Again, remove most of the clothing and sponge the body with water. Do not wipe it off but allow it to evaporate and thereby cool the body. Dehydration can be corrected by giving adequate fluid little and often and a great deal of nursing care may be needed. Burns to the skin will require dressing and treating and the risk of infection minimised. This can be a time-consuming exercise and requires a fair amount of skill. Again, the expedition nurse rises to the occasion!

Most cases of sunburn are minor but I have treated extensive burns to the shoulders of one young man. It took several days to sort out. It involved several nursing hours and much medical equipment and he was left in no doubt as to our feelings. I do not remember seeing another case of sunburn on that trip!

What do we do if someone is badly burnt?

Burns to the body can be divided into superficial burns and the deep. The former tend to be very painful as the nerves in the skin are not destroyed and associated with reddening of the skin and the formation of blisters. These heal on their own given time, providing they do not become infected. The latter are a different kettle of fish and tend not to be as painful as the nerves have been destroyed. These are full-thickness burns which do not heal on their own and need skin grafting. It is obvious that two types of burns can co-exist, but it is important to ascertain what types of burn may be present and the extent to which they both exist.

Burns are more likely to the hands and face but I suppose no part of the body is immune. If it is a hand or leg that is burnt, place the limb in cold water. This does two things; it relieves the pain and helps to promote healing. Having applied cold water to the burn wherever it may be, the next task is to clean the area, preferably with a sachet of sterile antiseptic or antiseptic creams or powders, depending on what you have available. I usually take an antibiotic impregnated gauze and apply this to the area. The wound is then dressed to prevent the area becoming infected. Antibiotics by mouth are not usually given but adequate pain relief must be obtained and in some situations the patient may need some form of sedation.

The vast majority of burns are minor but must be looked after carefully if they are to heal satisfactorily. The dressings will need to be changed on alternate days to start with and again an assessment of the type of burn is made. The area which is painless and not healing may well be a deep burn requiring attention on return home and may need skin grafting if it is to heal properly without scarring. In more extensive burns – heaven forbid – the patient may be shocked due to fluid loss and severe pain and need transporting to hospital where intravenous therapy in the form of saline and blood may be needed if the patient is to recover. I do not expect that you will have to cope with this eventuality!

Members are often not sure what to do with the blistering that occurs in superficial burns. I usually burst the blister with a sterile needle the plasma is allowed to drain away and then the burn is dressed. On no account peel away the dead skin as this protects the underlying healing skin, but apart from that it also makes the injury so much more painful. So allow the fluid to drain from the blister and then leave well alone. Nature is far more efficient than the hands of a meddling doctor or nurse!

What do we do if we think they are suffering from hypothermia?

In a cold environment the vessels in the skin vaso constrict and this reaction is followed by an increase in muscle tone and shivering. This helps the body to maintain and generate heat. Hypothermia is defined when the body temperature falls below 33 degrees centigrade. At first there is listlessness and confusion as the body temperature falls. Later loss of consciousness follows and death occurs due to heart failure from the direct action of the cold on the heart muscle. The heart usually fails as its rhythm becomes irregular and it is no longer capable of performing its task.

Hill walkers, climbers and skiers who are inadequately clothed in low temperatures are liable to develop hypothermia and also frostbite. This generally happens when people have become lost or immobilised due to adverse weather conditions or injury. The effects of hypothermia are accelerated by the use of alcohol so leave your brandy behind! The process of hypothermia on dry land proceeds relatively slowly and most victims recover by being placed in a well insulated sleeping bag. The temperature can also be increased by placing someone else in the same bag, so do be careful who you go away with! If the hypothermia is severe, additional warming aids may be used, for example, hot water bottles, but the practice of immersing the poor unfortunate patient in a bath of hot water is not be recommended. Rapid increase in body temperature can in itself be fatal as it has been associated with abnormal heart rhythms.

So the message is clear – do not venture forth without proper clothing. If you are unfortunate to be stranded by bad weather or injury do not rely on alcohol to revive your spirits and anyone who you may think has developed hypothermia must be kept warm by whatever means and help urgently summoned. Raise his body temperature slowly by sensible means and hopefully all will be well.

Not only does the mountaineer run the risk of developing hypothermia he is also at risk from frostbite due to local cooling of a limb and the freezing and death of body tissues. Frostbite is obvious, as hard white areas of skin on the extremities. As long as it involves only parts of the fingers, toes or hands it is best treated by thawing in water no hotter than the patient can stand without discomfort. The skin may turn black but then sloughs off leaving healthy tissue underneath.

Exposure in very cold climates can result in massive freezing of most of the tissues in a limb. In these cases slow warming is again mandatory, but if there has been extensive tissue destruction the surgeon may have his part to play.

The development of clothing for the mountaineer has helped

to reduce the incidence of cold injury for the mountaineer and it is foolhardy to venture forth without taking the proper precautions. Not only may you be putting your own life at risk but you also endanger the lives of the people who come to rescue you. So be prepared and be warned!

What to do if we think someone may have drowned?

Total immersion in water is followed by breath-holding for about five minutes and then massive inhalation of water in the lungs. In sea water drowning death is caused by cardiac arrest but in fresh water drowning the heart beats irregularly and then as it fails it stops beating. The immediate treatment of the victim without pulse or respiration is to clear the airway and start external cardiac massage and artificial respiration. If the doctor is carrying a gastric pump this should be passed as the stomach will be distended with water. He should also at the same time try to pass an endotracheal tube to maintain an airway. This may not obviously be possible if there is no doctor or he has not brought the necessary equipment with him.

Bring the unfortunate victim to the bank as soon as you can or to a firm surface, for example, a boat. First of all clear and maintain an airway by opening the mouth to remove any foreign matter and start artificial respiration. With the patient's neck slightly extended to open the airway, pinch his nose and by putting your mouth to his, forcibly breathe air into his lungs. Do this fifteen to twenty times a minute. If the heart has stopped beating it is no use doing this on its own and external cardiac massage has to be undertaken. Kneeling by the side of the patient and using the heal of your hand, start cardiac massage by pressing quite forcibly on the middle to lower part of the breast bone or sternum. You have then started the pump which will hopefully pump blood once again around the circulation. The rules are simple – ABC. A is for airway, B is for breathing and C is for circulation.

There are many organisations which teach first aid and if you are going to remote and potentially hostile environments it is your duty to learn about the resuscitation of an unconscious patient. It is not difficult, and even if you are not successful at least you will have tried.

What do we do if we think a wound needs suturing?

Wounds come in all shapes and sizes but fortunately most of them in my experience are small, requiring half a dozen sutures at the most. If a wound is gaping and bleeding badly the odds are it will need stitching. This is easy if a doctor is available but what do you do if there is not. First of all examine the wound and clean it using antiseptic sterile sachets. If it is small it may be possible to use skin or butterfly sutures. By pressing the edges together stick the skin suture across to enable the wound to heal. If it is larger and bleeding the first thing to do is to stop the bleeding by firm compression. Place a dressing over the wound and use either your hand or a belt – you compress the wound and the bleeding will stop. Once this has been achieved put a sterile dressing over the wound; if you have antibiotic impregnated gauze this may be used, or antibiotic powder or cream. It is important to try to stop the wound becoming infected. If you have stopped the bleeding, cleaned and dressed the wound there is nothing else you can reasonably do. If it is not possible to summon medical help the patient will come to no harm. He may be left with a scar, but at least the bleeding will have been stopped and the incidence of infection greatly reduced.

There may be an occasion when the bleeding will not stop and that raises the possibility of a bleeding artery. This is serious, but do not panic. Compress the wound as before and keep it compressed and then you have no other course of action but to transport the victim to hospital where he may need surgery to stop the bleeding.

Cuts and grazes and commonplace on expeditions and most of them heal without any problem. I usually, having cleaned them and dressed them, do no more. It is important to dress them to minimise the risk of infection. It is amazing where flies get to!

What do we do if we think someone has been bitten?

I suppose the first question is bitten or stung by what. Insect bites wasps and bees can be very painful but do not cause much hassle unless the bites are multiple. Insect bites are common but here again if you wander around in a state of undress you are asking for trouble. Bites should be dressed and again the risk of infection minimised. Going up the ladder, scorpion bites are next. In desert regions scorpions are common but seldom seen during the day. If you want to find them you only have to look under stones and you will not be disappointed. At night, however, they are a more common sight and it is important to wear suitable footwear. Walking around bare-footed is forbidden. If someone is bitten by a scorpion do not panic as although the bite is painful, it is not usually a threat to life. Tablets should be given to relieve the pain, for example, codeine phosphate, thirty milligrams, but if a doctor is at hand local anaesthetic can be infiltrated around the bite to relieve the pain. Here too, the bite should be dressed to prevent infection. Spider bites are also common and not likely to threaten life, although young children and the frail and elderly may be at risk. Bites from dogs and other mammals pose the risk of rabies. Members must be warned to stay away from dogs and not encouraged to approach them. It is not a question of, come here, nice little doggy! It is a question of staying well away from them. Rabies can be spread not only by being bitten but also from the lick of an infected animal. Rabies is a killer. I have gone into some length on snake bites and the warning is clear and simple. Use your common sense and stay clear. It is amazing how little heed is taken in respect of the risk of scorpion, spider and snake bites. Members of an expedition leave their sleeping bags open on the ground. As one young girl told me, she was only trying to air her sleeping bag by leaving it open on the ground. Shoes also pose a problem and they should be inspected before putting them on. This is another example of camp discipline which should not be neglected.

What do we do if someone has been badly injured?

If someone has been seriously injured in, for example, a rock fall or a road traffic accident and is lying still and obviously in a critical condition, the first assumption to make is that his life must be regarded as being in great danger. What can you do to help if you are in a remote place? First of all assume that he has broken a limb, may have internal injuries and may have a head injury. Try to assess the level of consciousness – does he respond to questioning. If he does then the likelihood is that he is not too badly hurt. If there is no response then he is in trouble. Try to assess the degree of damage and if he is conscious he will be able to tell you. – if not, you will have assume serious injury. Generally do not try to move him as if he has broken a limb he will experience great pain and movement may accelerate internal bleeding. Medical help must be summoned as a matter of urgency. If there is a doctor on the expedition send for him. I have mentioned before that when people go out they should only do so in groups of at least three. Someone must stay with the patient and the other summon help and guide the rescue party back. For the person left to look after the victim if he is unconscious the former must ensure that his airway is open, move him as little as possible and keep him warm. If he is able to swallow give him pain-relieving tablets, if you have them. There is little else you can do after that except hope that help comes as soon as possible.

If there is a doctor at hand it is his responsibility to resuscitate the patient, relieve his pain, be responsible for his evacuation from the scene and urgent admission to hospital. All doctors should carry airways, endotracheal tubes and tracheotomy tubes and at least have some knowledge as to how to use them or at least be prepared to have a go. Intravenous fluids including plasma expanders should be available, along with splints and a supply of morphine. When all this has been done the patient should be moved with great care onto a stretcher and carried to safety and that means hospital, wherever it may be.

It has to be pointed out to the members of an expedition that there are risks involved and, if relevant, the parents of the members should be informed as well. Not in a dramatic unreasonable way as to frighten them, but in a calm and sensible manner. There may be little you can do if there is serious injury on an expedition but that is also the case in this country where ambulance services are readily available and a hospital may be within easy reach. It is important that you have some knowledge of first aid and learn how to deal with an unconscious patient and at least have a go at mouth-to-mouth resuscitation and external cardiac massage. As I have said before, it is far better to have a go even if your attempts fail.

What should we do if someone has snow-blindness?

On snow-covered mountains and Polar regions sunburn is a common problem and particular care should be taken with the eyes in this aspect. The conjunctiva or membrane which protects the eye may be particularly sensitive to the sun's rays which in these circumstances may be severe, as they are both direct and reflected. If the eye is exposed to this risk the end result is snow-blindness. You will not be permanently blinded but you may be considerably incapacitated. As a result of such injury the eye becomes very painful, so much so that the eyelids go into spasm to protect the eye and you are left with a swollen, red and watering eye. Even on a cloudy day snow-blindness can occur. The condition is preventable by wearing suitable goggles or sunglasses. Your progress will be halted as you will not be able to see clearly and then run the risk of severe injury – for example, by falling, as your vision is seriously impaired. The treatment consists of being placed in the dark, the eyes prised open and local anaesthetic or steroid drops being instilled into the eye. It will take several days for you to recover and the eye has to be protected against further exposure to the sun which may mean bandaging the affected eye over. It usually does not cause permanent damage but you will not be very popular with your expedition leader. Like so many problems encountered in expedition medicine it is preventable by wearing suitable protection for the eyes.

I am often asked about sun-blocking creams and usually advise people just to cover up and not to use them, but in such circumstances sun blocking creams for your face and other exposed areas in Polar regions and on snow-covered mountains are necessary. In deserts you are better off wearing suitable clothing, including protective headgear.

ACUTE MOUNTAIN SICKNESS

This is a miserable and potentially dangerous condition and may lead to either or both of the following conditions – Acute Pulmonary Oedema and High Altitude Cerebral Oedema. Both these conditions may be insidious in onset but progress rapidly.

As the mountaineer climbs to high altitude he starts to have trouble breathing., becomes light headed, nauseated, and euphoric. This is followed by increasing lethargy and he becomes restless and may have trouble sleeping. The headache becomes worse, vomiting follows and he lapses into unconsciousness.

The expedition doctor must be on the lookout for early signs of this condition and when spotted should act immediately rather than waiting for other symptoms to develop. The mainstay of treatment is to urgently transfer the victim to a low altitude and both lasix and oxygen may well have to be administered.

This condition is preventable like most problems in Expedition Medicine and acclimatisation at lower levels is to be insisted on – so is the rate of ascent. It is no use being foolhardy as you may not just endanger your own life but you put at risk the rescuers who may have been summoned to bring you down to safety. The more remote the area you are travelling the more care has to be taken.

LOST IN A DESERT

The golden rule is usually to stay where you are and organise some form of signalling system. Collect everyone together, organise a camp and strictly ration all food and water. It is no use wandering off to find help if you do not know where help lies. If there is a village within walking distance it is reasonable to set off but in no other circumstances should the group be split up. The main problem for the expedition doctor is uncertainty and despair within his travelling companions.

Travelling in remote and potentially dangerous situations when trouble strikes I have never ceased to be impressed by the determination and resolution of young explorers. People caring for others, taking time to listen to the others problems and putting their own fears to the back of their minds for the time being. When you are in trouble it is important to sit down and carefully analyse the situation. Acting in haste and regretting it later is not to be encouraged. Formulate a constructive plan and most important of all try to keep to it. That day we were lost in the Chalbi desert we were not in any immediate danger. The main problem was fatigue and fear. It was more of a question of calming things down, making sure everyone knew what was going on and trying to lift morale. Panic is enemy number one in these difficult circumstances and a sense of humour helps to put things in their correct perspective.

WHAT SHOULD WE DO IF

Somebody has been eating my porridge

This is quite a common occurrence out in the bush. Food is not as plentiful as it is in Asda and animals and tribes may steal any unguarded fodder.

Firstly try and avoid the situation whereby your porridge can be easily taken from you. That is, don't make it too hot, hence having to go for a walk in the bush until it cools. This is a very silly thing to do and you would only have yourself to blame should your porridge disappear.

Secondly, lock all windows and doors, thus preventing

blonde little girls (aged between six and seven – usually from Germany) climbing in through the unlocked windows. You can, if you wish, leave your doors unlocked as it is highly unlikely that this child (that is, if it is a child) would walk in through a doorway (ask Hans Christian Anderson, if you wish).

Having taken these preventative steps, your porridge should be perfectly safe and alternative foods not needed. But PLEASE, PLEASE, PLEASE, if you do happen to see this little girl, do not under any circumstances approach her. She may be the child who steals the porridge, but, on the other hand, she could have got confused (being in the wrong place at the wrong time) and really be Red Riding Hood. If she does have the attire about her person, she may be being followed by Wil. E. Coyote-after her basket-who in turn will be in hot pursuit of a road runner, and, my oh my, things could really get tricky from here. You see each to their own! Everything in its place, as my mother said, but once cartoons, fairy stories and fables all intermingle, well, Lord knows what can happen. So you see, it is absolutely imperative that your porridge isn't too hot.

Now then, let's assume that your porridge HAS gone. Where do we go from here? Well, Asda is out, as we're in the bush. As is Tesco. So the best thing to do is order a Taxi (oh yes, primitive they may be but have you every known a black man to miss a fare). Once the taxi is at hand-everyone in and off to MacDonalds!

CONCLUSION

The responsibility of being an expedition doctor is not to be taken lightly. It is not an excuse for a holiday where little care is paid to the members with who you are travelling. It is a position of high responsibility and must be prepared carefully and thoughtfully from leaving home to returning to these shores. For it is here that the expedition finally ends.

Careful planning before you go is essential. Members must be aware of the risks that are involved and every care taken to minimise these. Discipline is the cornerstone of success not in a regimental attitude but with a sensible outlook and approach. Immunisations should be planned carefully, clothing and footwear must be appropriate, the preparation and serving of food observed and maintained and proper and correct behaviour and manners are not be underestimated. I am often asked about the more dramatic events relating to expedition medicine but always reply that it is my purpose to prevent such happenings! Prevention is far better than cure. There are times on the trip when you feel that there is nothing for you to deal with, especially in the early stages, but beware, do not let complacency take over because sooner or later something will happen and hopefully this will be out of your control and something you could not have anticipated.

It is important to keep your finger on the pulse of the expedition and to try and foretell what problems may arise and be in a position to deal with them. You must always try to be one step ahead. Looking after an expedition is comparable to looking after a family unit and this must come first in all situations that you find yourself in. You should be available at any time to anybody on the trip no matter what position they hold within the group to listen and help to sort out whatever problem they might have. I always go round at night to check with the various groups and, although it is usually a courtesy call, at least it makes people realise you are available and interested in their welfare. The problems are varied and not necessarily related to the expedition itself. Problems are often discussed that present themselves at home, whether it be education, work or domestic problems, and you should listen to these and offer sensible and constructive advice. It is amazing when in remote areas that you can think more clearly and develop more insight into problems that you have. It may be the first time people are able to come to terms with them and stuggle to sort them out.

I count myself fortunate to have been to some remote and beautiful places and looked after members on a trip and hopefully to help them enjoy it also. It brings great rewards and satisfaction, I hope that I have also helped people to face up to life in general and develop a more mature and understanding attitude to life. Some members set off in fear and trepidation and it is interesting to watch their self-confidence develop. Going on expeditions certainly helps to mould personalities; it gives you a much broader outlook on life and an understanding of the problems people face in different parts of the world.

If expeditions interest you my advice is to take the plunge and go. Expedition medicine is a fascinating branch of medicine, not without its risks but the rewards are enormous.